The Antonia Faizah Sinibaldi Story

Strength, Hope, and Perseverance

HOLLYROCK ✦ MILLER
MARKETING COMMUNICATIONS

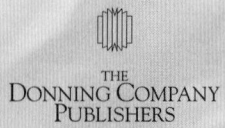

THE
DONNING COMPANY
PUBLISHERS

The Antonia Faizah Sinibaldi Story

Strength, Hope, and Perseverance

By Antonia Sinibaldi with Andrew Frothingham

Copyright © 2017 by Hollyrock/Miller
Produced by Hollyrock/Miller Marketing Communications

All rights reserved, including the right to reproduce this work in any form whatsoever without permission in writing from the publisher, except for brief passages in connection with a review. For information, please write:

The Donning Company Publishers
731 S. Brunswick
Brookfield, MO 64628

Lex Cavanah, General Manager
Nathan Stufflebean, Production Supervisor
Pamela Koch, Senior Editor
Terry Epps, Graphic Designer
Katie Gardner, Marketing & Production Coordinator

Mike Mannicci, Project Director

Cataloging-in-Publication Data

Names: Sinibaldi, Antonia, 1997- author. | Frothingham, Andrew, author.
Title: The Antonia Faizah Sinibaldi story : strength, hope, and perseverance
   / by Antonia Sinibaldi with Andrew Frothingham.
Description: Brookfield, MO : The Donning Company Publishers, [2017]
Identifiers: LCCN 2016055139 | ISBN 9781681841007 (hard cover : alk. paper)
Subjects: LCSH: Sinibaldi, Antonia -- Health. | Quadriplegics--Biography. |
   Spinal cord--Wounds and injuries--Patients--Biography.
Classification: LCC RC406.Q33 S56 2017 | DDC 617.4/82044092 [B] --dc23
LC record available at https://lccn.loc.gov/2016055139

Printed in the United States of America at Walsworth

Dedication

I dedicate this book to my grandparents and the rest of my family and friends.

CONTENTS

8 — Preface
9 — Acknowledgments

11 — **Chapter 1:** Crash
13 — **Chapter 2:** BC (Before Crash)
      Mom
17 — **Chapter 3:** The Accident
19 — **Chapter 4:** Changed Forever
21 — **Chapter 5:** Blythedale
23 — **Chapter 6:** Cliffside Park
25 — **Chapter 7:** Rehab at Home
      Alek Kalmus
29 — **Chapter 8:** Lawsuit
      Dave Mazie, Esq.
      Dave Freeman, Esq.
33 — **Chapter 9:** Faith
35 — **Chapter 10:** Music!
37 — **Chapter 11:** Dance
39 — **Chapter 12:** School
41 — **Chapter 13:** Spasms
43 — **Chapter 14:** Temperature
45 — **Chapter 15:** Fourth Grade
47 — **Chapter 16:** Camp Friends
49 — **Chapter 17:** Mother
51 — **Chapter 18:** Father
53 — **Chapter 19:** Settlement
      Wade Martin
55 — **Chapter 20:** Weehawken
      Antonia Valicenti
57 — **Chapter 21:** Performing Arts/Music
      Brad Mehrten
61 — **Chapter 22:** Anchor

63 — **Chapter 23:** Brother
   Jib
97 — **Chapter 24:** Inspiration
   Hugh Miller
99 — **Chapter 25:** Performing
101 — **Chapter 26:** Technology
   Andrew Purwin, technology consultant
107 — **Chapter 27:** Neighbors
109 — **Chapter 28:** Friends
   Ashley Acevedo
111 — **Chapter 29:** Love
113 — **Chapter 30:** Mental Illness
115 — **Chapter 31:** Sadness
117 — **Chapter 32:** PTSD
119 — **Chapter 33:** High School
   Rob Ferullo
123 — **Chapter 34:** Two Proms!
125 — **Chapter 35:** Finding the Right College
127 — **Chapter 36:** Ongoing Challenges
129 — **Chapter 37:** Taking Control
131 — **Chapter 38:** Hope
133 — **Chapter 39:** Find Inspiration
135 — **Chapter 40:** Learn to Accept Help
137 — **Chapter 41:** Believe in Something Bigger than Yourself
139 — **Chapter 42:** Never Give Up
141 — **Chapter 43:** Be Different
143 — **Chapter 44:** Speak Up
145 — **Chapter 45:** Perspective
147 — **Chapter 46:** Heroes
149 — **Chapter 47:** Invitation: Ask Me!
151 — **Chapter 48:** Who Am I?
153 — **Chapter 49:** Why Did I Write This Book?
155 — **Chapter 50:** How Did I Write This Book?
157 — **Chapter 51:** Forgiving
159 — **Chapter 52:** My Destiny

PREFACE

Have you ever lost a life and been reawakened to a new one? You know, that "pinch-me" moment where you ask yourself, "Is this my life right now?" If you have, then you will understand what you're about to read. If you haven't, my story will be an eye-opener for you. Either way, you should never take life for granted because one day you might wake up and long for the days when you thought you were so miserable before.

Life changes in a blink of an eye. It did for me. And it is still doing it to this day, to the point where I'm always asking, "Is this real?"

When I'm alone, I constantly ponder about everything that I have been through. I have so many questions.

"Why me?"

"What's the future going to be like for me?"

"Will it ever change?"

After asking those questions and more for a long time, I understand that while I may never find all the answers, I have learned a bit from the experiences that I have been through. While I have not, and may never, reached a state of full acceptance of what's happened, I have resolved to make the best of my situation by sharing my story in the hope that it might help others dealing with injuries, mental illness, and other challenges.

I do this as much for me as I do for others. I devoutly wish to be understood. I need to be heard. That's why I write in my own voice, not in fancy, flowery language. I want you to know the real me.

ACKNOWLEDGMENTS

This is my book. I am responsible for everything in it. However, I couldn't have created and produced it without the help of many people, several of whom you will hear from in the book.

I want to acknowledge, in particular, the assistance of:

- Andrew Frothingham, who helped me organize the contents of the book.
- Hugh Miller and his team at Hollyrock/Miller who handled the production of the book.
- My mother, my brother, and my family and friends who supported me while writing this book and listened to me patiently (for the most part) as I developed the themes and ideas in this book.

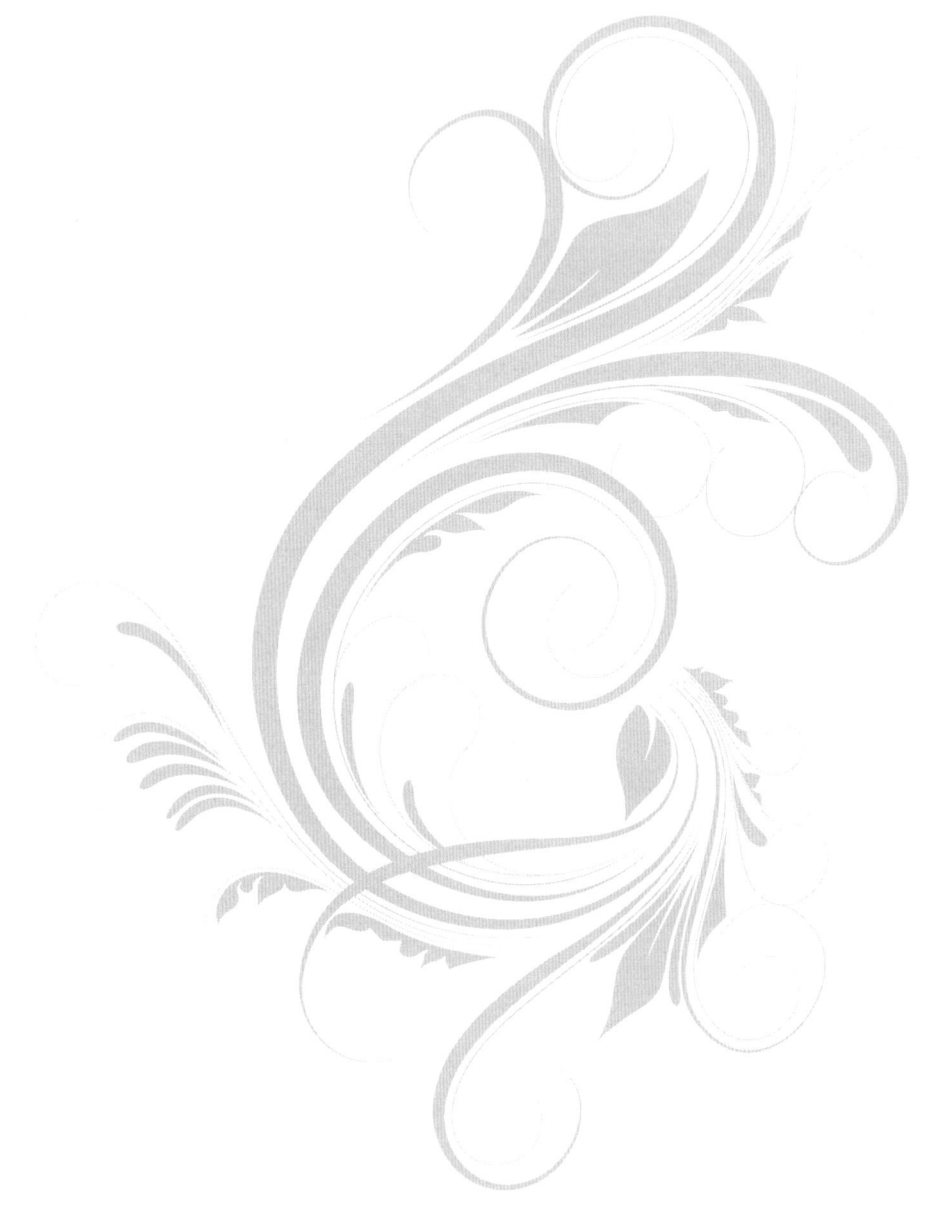

Chapter 1
Crash

Everything was right. I was just over two years old and I was safe and secure in my mother's arms. My father, my mother, and I were in one of our favorite places, our car. We were coming back from a fun, seasonal outing, headed for home. The car's warmth surrounded all of us, and my parents' happiness and love surrounded me. All was right in my world. The road and a bright future seemed to unfurl before us.

Then, suddenly, there was noise, impacts, shattered glass, torn metal, broken bodies. And pain, incredible pain. All the light that had been in my world was extinguished as darkness rushed in. I slipped in and out of consciousness with little idea of what was being done to me or where I was.

When I finally regained full consciousness, the world felt completely different. Nothing was right. There was no longer a way forward. Maybe not even hope or a future. That's when my real journey began.

Chapter 2
BC (Before Crash)

To understand my story, we have to go so far back down memory lane that we go past my genuine, personal memories and to the stories that I've been told about my birth and early childhood.

I was born on June 21, 1997. I am my parents' elder child and the youngest girl on both the Italian and the Guyanese sides of my family. When I came home from the hospital, my father surrounded me with 1,000 roses. One of my uncles took a series of pictures of this extravagant gesture. I have looked at them countless times. There I am, a tiny baby wrapped up snugly at the center of a sea of flowers. Some of the pictures include my mother looking lovely and younger than I can ever remember her being. My father shows up beaming with pride, radiating optimism, and loaded with youthful energy. This is the start of my personal mythology. It's a time and a world where everything looks, literally, rosy.

According to my mother, my personality as a baby was similar to the best parts of my personality today. I was, and still can be, very outgoing. I was a very mischievous, but loving, baby girl. I would constantly play with my grandmother by hiding her glasses. At the time, living with us were my grandma, my grandpa, and two of my mom's brothers. I would go up into my uncles' apartment and constantly mess around and steal their items, including chocolates.

Even then, I wasn't shy about speaking up when I knew what I wanted. One of my uncles still likes to tease me with the phrase "last time, Mommy, last time." That's what I would say when I was bouncing on the beds on the third floor and didn't want to go downstairs and go to bed. He claims that I would try to get away with saying this as many times as I could.

At that age, I also demonstrated a love for motion. I would go in front of the mirror and randomly start dancing. (It seems like some things never change:

I still love dancing, just in a slightly different way.) I would say to my mom, "dance, Mommy, dance."

When I was a baby, my grandparents would babysit me while my parents and uncles would work. I would stay up waiting until my mom came home. She didn't arrive until around 9 pm, but, despite the late hour, I always insisted that it was *"Spend Time with Me Time."* I would beg her to read to me or take me to the park. *What can I say? I couldn't get attention from her during the day, so I demanded it at night.*

According to my parents, we started traveling when I was about a year-and-a-half old. We looked for opportunities to add Fridays and/or Mondays onto weekends so we could go on longer and longer family trips. My father loved to drive, and long distances were no problem at all. We went as far as the Thousand Islands on the New York/Canada border. Once when my parents could arrange an even longer stretch of time off, we drove to Florida. When my parents couldn't attach extra days onto a weekend, we still took road trips, although some of them took us no farther than New York City. One of the times he took me there, we went to a museum that had a chandelier. When I saw it, I started singing "Happy Birthday" because I thought it was a birthday cake.

Often trips were planned so I could be shown off to relatives or friends (mostly family).

Aside from a tendency to get carsick, I was a good traveler. I was a friendly baby, and I would say "hi' to everyone, including random people who would pass by. Life was good, happy, and peaceful. Unfortunately, this happy period did not last very long.

Mom

"Antonia always wants to learn, to do more, and to do anything anyone else can. She was born with that spirit.

I have always treated her as if she were not in a wheelchair. After all, she was born normal and healthy, and despite all the hardships she has gone through, she still is the same person.

Antonia and I get a lot of strength and support from our religious beliefs. I grew up in a very religious home, and I read the Quran. It helps you look at things in a very positive way. Antonia and I each embrace the idea that there is a plan for us. That helps us go forward.

Rather than worry, which won't change what will happen, we make the best of the circumstances we find ourselves in. That doesn't mean we are passive. Just the opposite: I will speak up for Antonia when needed, although she's quite good at speaking up for herself now.

Our family life is not exactly what I might have envisioned when I was young. For example, because of all the assistance that Antonia needs, we have had more people around and our lives have been more public. On weekends, I try not to have help other than relatives. I view this as family time. It's when we get to experience a greater measure of privacy, quiet and peace."

Chapter 3
The Accident

Another series of pictures that I have looked at many times was taken on October 24, 1999, the day our real journey began; the day our lives changed forever. My parents had decided that we should go on a family outing to New Hope, Pennsylvania, where we rode on a quaint, restored, steam train and picked pumpkins in anticipation of Halloween, which was only a week away. At the time the photos were taken, we were a happy family without a care in the world. But by the time these photos were developed, *our world had gone to hell and back.*

Our drive back home started well enough. But once we were in New Jersey, a drunk driver rammed his truck head-on into our car. The drunk driver who hit us had hit two other vehicles before us. *"Third time's the charm," as they say — we were the ones most severely hurt.*

The driver had been coming back from a Giants football game at what was then known as Giants Stadium. Unfortunately, he thought it was "OK" to drink fourteen beers and smoke marijuana before getting behind the wheel of his truck. According to my dad, who was the driver of our car, everything happened so fast that "my life flashed before my eyes."

I barely survived the accident. In fact, technically I died and was revived twice. *What can I say? It wasn't meant for me to leave this messed-up planet.* I was a two-year-old girl who suffered and still suffers with a C2 to C5 incomplete spinal cord injury. From then on, I became a quadriplegic. I am unable to control any movement below my neck. I cannot breathe on my own and depend on assistance from a ventilator 24/7. A machine, my "vent," pumps 95 percent of the air I breathe in and out of my lungs. The doctors, then and now, have never seen a baby survive an injury like that. *I always knew I was special and one in a million.*

Thank God, my mother was not as physically injured as I was, although she did sustain injuries severe enough to put her into a coma for about a week. My father was not physically injured, but the collision clearly had a massive impact on him. Learning that his daughter and wife were severely injured was not easy for him, or for our family. The worst part for him was learning that their baby girl would need assistance twenty-four hours a day for the rest of her life. This was not easy for him to accept.

While my mother was recovering, my father stayed by my side through everything. It drove him crazy to see me not getting the treatment I needed. The hospital where I was first treated could only do so much for me. They were not capable of meeting my needs. Once my mom was stable enough for rehab, she told my dad that I should be moved to a better equipped and staffed hospital, preferably someplace close to where she would be for rehab. That is exactly what they did.

Chapter 4
Changed Forever

According to my parents, I was transferred from a hospital here in New Jersey to, at the time, one of the best hospitals in New York. My mom's rehab wasn't too far from the hospital I was in and was also close enough to where I went for rehab. My dad still stood by my side, slept on the floor, and did whatever he could to make me as comfortable as possible. I would say "ice, ice, Daddy, Daddy, ice" (<u>not</u> *the Vanilla Ice song "Ice, Ice Baby"; I was making a real request*), and he would give me ice chips as often as he could. Now that I am older, I understand that, because of being newly injured at the time, while I could not sense room temperature, inside I felt heat.

I have a tracheostomy (the hole in my windpipe, which is also known as the trachea, where my vent is attached — often called a "trach") and had a gastrostomy tube (also known as a feeding tube or a g-tube). At some point, the doctors wanted to see if by any chance I could swallow and tolerate food . . . *granted, if you've ever been in a hospital then you know that "tolerate" isn't exactly the word I should be using here, but anyway . . .* All the doctors were shocked and pleased that I was able to speak and swallow with the trach and the g-tube. The ice chips were also part of the test to see if I could handle swallowing food. My g-tube fortunately came out on its own one night in 2004, and my parents and I agreed that if I could eat and swallow, there was no need for it to be put back in. The doctors agreed. I am so happy I can eat and drink like a "normal" person. I love food, and I have a fairly decent appetite. I am forever grateful for these abilities.

My body, my situation, and my life are fundamentally different from that of a typical person. Most people only have to think about their breathing when they are taking a yoga class or singing professionally (*or after someone talks about thinking about breathing*). I have to think about my breathing all the time. I can't breathe on my own. A typical person's breathing automatically slows down when they sleep and speeds up when they are awake. That doesn't happen for me. I have to change the settings on my vent in order to sleep at night, and change them again when I get up. I sometimes change the settings on my vent when I have a voice lesson or performance so I have the extra strength and air I'll need.

If I'm arching (spasming) and my muscles are really tight, you might hear me ask whoever is caring for me to disconnect my vent and use "Ambu," a manual method of pumping air into the lungs. (Technically, AMBU stands for Artificial Manual Breathing Unit.) It provides a stronger and faster breath than the vent.

When typical people go to sleep, they lie down and unconsciously get into a comfortable position. I have to have my mom or whoever is taking care of me rearrange my body so that I am in a position that my body will like in order to not spasm. In fact, I had to develop and learn a particular position. No one taught me. Perhaps they couldn't because this posture reflects my unique body dynamics.

A person can have a pretty simple experience of room temperature. Except for drafts, the room either feels too hot, too cold, or comfortable. But, my injury has messed up my body's ability to sense and adjust to temperature. Different parts of my body feel temperature differently. When the air feels comfortable on my face, I will not feel it on my legs, which for the most part only feel extreme temperature. Basically, the farther away a body part is from my head, the less it can sense temperature. Even if I felt a consistent temperature in all parts of my body, I would not feel the same way that a typical person does at the same temperature. In a room where the temperature is 70 degrees, most people will feel comfortable; I'll feel chilled, the way a typical person would in a 59-degree room.

Chapter 5
Blythedale

The next stop on my recovery journey was rehab. *No, not the Amy Winehouse rehab.* I spent a year at what is still one of the best children's rehabilitation centers, especially for brain and spinal cord injuries, Blythedale Hospital in Valhalla, New York. The team of medical professionals were amazing. Blythedale is where I have my earliest and clearest childhood memories. They are all good memories. I'm sure that it doesn't hurt that while I was there, my mom completed her rehab and was now, as far as I was concerned, all better.

Believe it or not, Blythedale was a recovery paradise for children. At Blythedale, I felt like a kid. My medical needs did not bother me. Around the entrance they had characters from shows that all little children enjoyed. For example, they had a castle with Barney and Baby Bop. There was a playroom where families could interact with other patients and their families. They had a beautiful piano that I fell in love with. If I remember correctly, my cousin and I would play with it, and the feeling of hearing music made me feel well enough to ask somebody to hold my hand and let me touch the keys. That was before the extreme sensation came in. I was gaining feeling but not in a painful way. Now when we as a family discuss it, they are shocked I remember because I was so young and fragile at the time. I guess that was another early sign of my passion for the performing arts.

The physical and occupational therapists at Blythedale were amazing. In fact, they were the ones who helped me get my first power chair and my first stander. I have so many good memories, but my favorite has to be the one where I drove my power chair for the very first time. The first time I drove my chair, this overwhelming feeling came over me; I was unsure what the feeling was at first. The feeling was freedom. I was free, if only for a little while, from depending on someone. I was able to control the chair ALL BY MYSELF! I still feel free when I drive my chair. It gives me a feeling of independence that's good for my mind. Being able to drive myself in certain situations eases some of the anxiety that I feel. We will get to that part later.

I'm lucky to have some good photographs that I can look at to confirm that my memories are accurate. In every photo taken of me at Blythedale I'm smiling.

Chapter 6
Cliffside Park

After almost an entire year . . . finally it was time to go home. The sad part was that the girl who had left one year before was not the girl who returned. When I came home, I was three, and this is when I started understanding what my life would be from now on. I was trying to be a little girl although it was hard because I was still learning my *new body*. At the time, I could not lie on my stomach, I could not feel my legs unless they were spasming or someone was putting pressure on them, my fingers would constantly feel like cold needles, and my vision would go in and out of being blurry.

In Cliffside Park, I slept on the second floor but spent a lot of the day on the first floor. My parents would carry me and my vent up the stairs.

Soon, my mom was healthy enough to go back to work, so for the most part it was my dad, my grandma, and I.

A few years later, when my dad wasn't around, my mother would put the vent on her back and then pick me up and take me up the stairs by herself. Back then my mother was younger and I was smaller, but it was, nonetheless, an indication of the amazing strength and devotion that she still has.

Chapter 7
Rehab at Home

Being home wasn't all that easy because this is when physical therapy, occupational therapy, and chiropractic treatment came into my life. Most of those services were paid for by Cliffside Park, the town that I then lived in. The town also built my first ramp.

Going through all that therapy was not easy; it was painful. I was exercising or being exercised at a level that I wasn't ready for. At the same time, I was regaining feeling in some parts of my body. The problem was that I was newly injured, but I was being treated like a person who had already had ample time to adjust to their injury. The therapists did not understand my condition and did not even seem to try to understand. I would be crying because of the extreme pain, and nobody would listen to me. My grandmother would get mad, and she would say to the physical and occupational therapists, "Go easy on her. She's new to this. Can't you hear she's saying it's too much?"

Around this time I started receiving nursing care and trying to get used to having all these people around me. *I'm grateful for everybody who helps me, but the older I get, the more annoying and frustrating it gets.* The nurses I had were not up to the standards that we had come to expect at Blythedale. My father would get angry with them if they mistreated me, *and, believe me, they did.* I have many stories about this that I could tell.

The pain I experienced wasn't all physical. I felt like I was trapped in a glass cage of emotion. The nurses in the beginning would constantly make numerous mistakes, which made my father mad. For example, one of them overfed me when she should have known that I needed time to digest. I was too young to know what was too much feeding from the feeding pump. Another nurse did not check the milk in the bag until my dad did and realized that there were ants inside of it. *(Yes, ANTS!)* I have so many stories to tell, but, realistically, there are not enough pages in this book to tell you half the crap we've been through.

I like to be positive whenever I can, so I'd like to shine a light on one very positive development that happened during this period of time: I met Aleksander Kalmus. Alek is a gifted chiropractor. Once he started working with me, it soon became clear that in addition to understanding my physical challenges, he also understood me as a person more than anyone else. We are still friends, and I still use him. He takes the time to listen and work with my body. That is why I have kept him for so long. As I age and my body changes, he works with us to find new ways to address whatever new tightness and pains I experience. He continues to be interested in and really understand my perspectives on the world. He and I are so simpatico that we communicate quickly and easily. Our conversations are creative; they nourish my brain and soul.

Alek Kalmus

"I have known Antonia for years. I worked with her when she was very young, soon after her accident. We lost contact for several years, only to reconnect when she was thirteen. One of my first impressions was 'this young child is a fighter. She has a strong will to live.' She still has that will today. That's a good thing because she has so many issues she has to fight every day. Everything she does requires energy. Sometimes, she is exhausted and has a bad day, which is to be expected.

Another thing that has remained the same over the years is the strength of her bond with her mother, Fazila. Antonia probably learned much of her determination from her mother. Fazila is, by nature, a bit stoic. I think Antonia learned this, too. Antonia is more vocal about her pains and challenges because she has to be. But she also bears a lot of things in silence.

Together, they are ready to question any limitation and work to improve. Many people would have just accepted the doctor's word when they were told that Antonia would always be 100 percent dependent on the vent. Not these two. They have had the courage to experiment with disconnecting the vent in order to stimulate and build her muscles.

Antonia and her mother are both keen observers. I appreciate that because I, too, am an observer. In Antonia's case, there may be a downside to her always-active intelligence. Antonia doesn't get to devote as much of her time and energy to physical tasks as most of us do; as a result, she has much more mental time. She spends a great deal of time analyzing and speculating about herself. Sometimes, she speculates about whether or not her thoughts and feelings are 'healthy.' My sense is that her reactions are, pretty much, those of a normal person faced with extraordinary circumstances and equipped with unusual awareness and insight into herself.

Working with Antonia tends to be a rich, rewarding experience because she brings so much humor, character, and frankness to every situation. She and her mother continue to inspire me."

Chapter 8
Lawsuit

I'm blessed. While I was focused on my own health and emotions, as was natural for a child of my age, various adults were hard at work on my behalf. My mother and father were deeply involved in all this, but at the time I was too young to understand what was going on. I'm not sure of all of the steps they went through and how it all happened, but somehow they connected with Dave Mazie and Dave Freeman, fantastic lawyers who became passionate about my case, as well as family friends. I received a settlement that helps me with the extraordinary costs I face as a result of my injury.

Dave Mazie, Esq.

"Antonia never ceases to amaze me. I'm not sure how many good days most people in her situation would have, but as far as I can tell, Antonia never has a bad day. She's nothing short of incredible.

At the trial, the other side asked for a smaller settlement using the argument that Antonia might not live very long. But there were no statistics available about length of life for people who have experienced a spinal cord injury like hers at such a young age.

When she testified at the trial, she told the courtroom that she wanted to be a singer or a ballerina. Everyone in the room knew that these things would be impossible for Antonia, and that's what made the testimony so moving — her positivity in the face of her injuries.

When her case was settled, it was international news. We had a big press conference. Antonia was the star, and she sang a song for the reporters and cameramen. When she was finished, everyone there broke out in applause. I was later told that reporters aren't supposed to react to those being interviewed, but this was such a special case that they couldn't help themselves.

In high school, Antonia was a part of a mock trial competition, and she asked me to be the trial coach for her school's team. She was amazing. She played the part of a witness, which meant she had to respond to both direct examination and to cross-examination. This is tough to start with, and Antonia was doing it without the ability to breathe on her own, without the ability to move below her neck, and without the ability to hold up paper with notes. She even had to make it through some spasming. She did so well that after the competition students from other teams came up and introduced themselves, telling her that she was an inspiration to them.

There is nothing more rewarding than being able to help someone like Antonia. I was able to help change her life, and I expect that she, in turn, will help others. I can see her using her magnetic personality as an advocate around the issue of drunk driving or spinal cord injuries."

Dave Freeman, Esq.

"I went to Antonia's high school graduation. To start with, it was amazing that she was able to graduate. I got the sense that all of her classmates and all of her teachers loved her. I can't think of another client whose graduation I attended. That's not surprising. Things having to do with Antonia are often exceptional.

Antonia has no cognitive impairment, despite the severity and extent of the injuries she suffered. That's exceptional.

Her presence has always been exceptional. Antonia testified at the trial concerning the accident she was in. She was only seven years old. She was very pleasant and charming. With no prompting from any of us, she just started singing in front of the jury. She stole everyone's heart.

The publicity surrounding her case moderated alcohol sales at sport venues across the country. Today, almost everywhere, there are two-drink limits, everyone is IDed, vendors are careful not to serve someone who shows signs of already having over-indulged, and they stop serving alcohol earlier in the game.

I'm delighted to have Antonia and her mother as friends. They are special. I think that Antonia gets a lot of her drive from Fazila. After all, when they still lived in Cliffside Park, her mom would carry her and her vent up and down the stairs every day.

Antonia and Fazila are beautiful people — very inspirational. They want to contribute despite their circumstances. They want to be out there helping others. I know they help me. Antonia always has a smile on her face, and when I think of her, I smile, too."

Chapter 9
Faith

When I was a little kid, while my mom was working, her mother — my grandmother — would commute from her home in New York to our home in New Jersey to help out. She is the one who introduced me to Islam. This became a source of inspiration and light with the help of my grandmother, not just physically, but spiritually as well. My mom came from a very religious Islamic Guyanese family, and the two most religious people in it were my grandparents.

My grandparents were naturally concerned about my health, so they would always say prayers over me. My grandmother would teach me my prayers, or surahs, and if I couldn't pronounce or remember them, she would sing them. This helped me to remember them. As I learned my first few prayers and as my grandmother discovered that I could sing, she would say, "Alhamdulillah (which means "glory to Allah" in Arabic), Baba, you have a gift."

Of all the people in my family, my grandfather was always the most religious. He would hold my cheeks and pray. He would also tell me the same story over and over again, "Ahh, Baba, you would jump on grandpa's bed and run straight to grandma." My grandparents would call me "Baba" and "Bettie," words used in Arabic when speaking fondly to babies or small children. *Today, I wish I could hear their words again.*

Thanks to my grandparents who brought Islam into my life, now that I am older I can teach myself; and my mom continues to teach my brother and me, too. I am grateful for what my grandmother taught me and for what my grandfather demonstrated — when I hear certain prayers, they remind me of him. Being raised in an Islamic family makes me the beautiful young lady that I am striving to be. It teaches me to respect my elders *(or at least try to respect them)*. It gives me peace with my mind *(we will talk about my mind later)*. Most of all, I feel close to my grandparents. I feel like when I try to be the best version of a Muslim while being myself, I'm doing part of what Allah wants me to be doing. I know that my grandma and grandpa are definitely proud of me. Islam is a great way to give you inner peace, and it is not just a religion; it is a way of life. Life has many different features, and everybody on this planet has many different beliefs, but one of my favorite quotes from the Quran is "and we created you into different nations and different tribes so that you may get to know one another." This quote, basically, is my motto, and I was raised to try to be respectful to everyone around me. *It may be hard as hell, but in the end, it's worth it.*

Chapter 10
Music!

Music! Music officially came into my life, and Alhamdulillah, it is by far the best gift I ever had. I was five years old when I fell in love with music and singing, thanks to my grandma and my dad. As I mentioned earlier, Grandma introduced me to music through prayer and nursery rhymes. My dad was also one of my biggest musical influences; sometimes he still is. I remember him showing me *The Sound of Music*, which is by far my favorite musical. He would also play old classics like Frank Sinatra, Frankie Valli and the Four Seasons, The Carpenters, The Rolling Stones, The Eagles, The Beatles, and so much more. I memorized almost every song in *The Sound of Music* when I was only five years old.

I was in a special education pre-K for two years, and one of the classes I had to take was speech therapy. One of the exercises I remember was having to say something to a recorder, play it back, then learn from it. I asked my teacher if I could sing instead of talking, and that is what I did. I sang "Do-Re-Mi" ("Doe, a deer") from *The Sound of Music* in front of the whole class.

For the most part, I have very dark and painful memories of my first few years in school, but this is one of the better ones. I felt proud of myself because I showed everyone that I am not just a quadriplegic; I am much more than that. Nobody understood my condition, and if I remember correctly, they were speechless after I sang. It felt good to show them who I really am, not just another patient. I'm a person who has feelings just like any other person on this planet, but I felt like they didn't think that.

Today I am a young adult, and I have so many musical influences from my mom and dad and today's generation that it helps me make my own music. I constantly write songs. When I'm not writing and I'm listening to music, I imagine myself singing it. I even imagine myself playing my two favorite instruments *(other than my voice, of course)*: the piano and the guitar. I may not have the ability to play an instrument, but my ability to hear has grown over the years, and I can tell when a note is slightly off. I am also a perfectionist when it comes to my own music, and I write from the heart. I don't know what my life would be like if I didn't have the gift of singing. Even when I'm not singing, I can feel the music. *Exception: Later in this book, I reveal that I suffer from depression. When my depression is really bad, I don't feel the music; my life is empty.*

Chapter 11
Dance

The first few years I have really good memories of my dad. I remember every morning he would say, "Buon giorno" to us, and to me, his little girl, he would say, "Ciao bella" in a deeply musical voice. He said to me, "You have such a beautiful voice." That is when I fell in love with singing. At home, we would also dance. Daddy would pick me up out of the chair or move my chair around the room, and whoever was there would follow with the vent stand. In my diary that I was writing in at the time, I would say that I wanted to be a ballerina. We would dance to Fred Astaire and Ginger Rogers, The Beatles, and *Dirty Dancing*. In grades pre-K through second, they had father-daughter dances, and we would go each time. Dancing with my dad for the first few years inspired me even more to want to perform. It gave me this feeling that I have a voice and I can move, too, just in a different way. I am absolutely not afraid of driving my chair and dancing. I love inspiring people in many ways, and dancing with my chair is one of the ways. I love to party, and I am at that age where any party where there is music and dancing is where I want to be.

Chapter 12
School

Cliffside Park, New Jersey, was the town that I was raised in from birth to eleven years old. I started out in a special education pre-K classroom. It was not a great start for me, but because of my injury, I had to start off somewhere. The program and I were not a great match. If it weren't for my dad, I probably would have been homeschooled. He petitioned the town to allow me to physically go to school instead of the staff coming to my home. I was happy and excited when I first found out that I was going to school because at that young age the injury was all I ever knew, so I figured all the kids would look like me. However, it was more challenging than I thought.

Each student whether in special or regular education has different needs, but mine were the most severe. I remember when I was five, during a physical therapy session, I had to be placed on my stomach. I was a newly injured patient, and they were treating me like a long-term injured patient. My teacher was mad at me. I told her, "I can't breathe on my stomach." My body couldn't handle the pressure of what they were doing to me, and I started to cry and kept complaining that I couldn't breathe. The nurse that I had at the time was the longest-serving nurse I ever had. I still love her like a second mother, but back then she was new to this, like I was, and did not know how to react. *As you can read later on, this period of time is when I started to experience depression, anxiety, and Post-Traumatic Stress Disorder (PTSD) because I thought that everything was my fault.*

As the years went on, all of us were learning from each other and from the teachers, physical therapists (PTs), occupational therapists (OTs), and my nurse. Depending on which teacher, *and this goes for everyone in general,* you need to work with me, and I will work with you. Not every grade was bad. What made things bad were communication issues and when my muscle spasms started coming out. When the spasms started coming and I started crying, I was kicked out of class because, at first, I wasn't listening to my nurse (*because back then it was even more of a one-way street*). I had other teachers and therapists who would yell at me for my spasms and for crying and disagreeing. *Everything the nurse and therapists said was accepted as automatically correct.* As the years went on, she and I gained an understanding that the person who knows my body best is . . . me. *(Surprise!)* This is when our relationship got really close, and I hope it will continue to grow. This is something that everybody who works with me has to appreciate. I'm not rude. I'm not selfish, and if you work with me, I'll work with you.

Chapter 13
Spasms

As time moved on, as it tends to, suddenly I was seven, and one of my trips to hell started. MUSCLE SPASMS! Spasms can be caused by a number of different things. Ever since the accident, during the first few years, my body was numb, but I would suffer from overheating, blotchiness, congestion, high blood pressure, etc. Doctors refer to this as autonomic dysreflexia. From two to seven years old, I wouldn't spasm because of this. However, now this can trigger spasming, but not all the time.

The new spasms were not generally triggered that way. For five years, I had been regaining feeling in my body. By the time I turned seven, I had gained near complete feeling. *Maybe too much feeling.* For most able-bodied people, their sensations of touch, noise, movement, etc., do not affect them the same way they do a person with neurological damage. At the time, my body was so sensitive that anything would set it off into a SEVERE MUSCLE SPASM. In other words, now all sorts of external stimuli could trigger spasms. This made it hard to go to school, change position, and have too many people around.

For those of you lucky enough not to suffer from spasms, let me tell you what they are like. When you have a spasm, it's as if something in your body has short-circuited and sent a signal to some muscles telling them to go crazy. This is not a voluntary thing. I don't think it's possible to intentionally spasm, and if it were, I can't imagine why anyone would do it. A spasm can often tighten a muscle up so much that it hurts more than a cramp. It can get so tight that it is as if somebody is squeezing me. This is when you would hear me say, "Ambu." Just to recap . . . Ambu is a hand-operated device that pumps a strong breath of air into my lungs. When my spasms get painful and my muscles get tight past a certain point, my vent doesn't provide enough air and I don't have the strength to pull it in. I need someone to pump in the greater amount of air that my system needs to stabilize itself.

The first few years, on the pain scale, my pain was always a ten and beyond. On top of the pain, having a bunch of muscles being triggered in rapid succession is exhausting. Not to mention the weirdness for you and all those around you of having some of your muscles seem to develop minds of their own.

Lots of different parts of my body can have different sensations. The more sensitive a certain part can be or can get, the more likely it will cause a spasm. Sometimes if I am very sensitive, I can control my body to an extent and delay the spasm for a certain amount of time by breathing slowly with the help of medication, meditation, and distraction. However, if I lived in a perfect world, this would work all the time. The spasms that I hate most involve my back muscles and can cause me to arch so badly. If any of my spasms are not under control, they can leave me in extreme pain. It's as if I were a marionette and some sadistic puppeteer was trying to see if I could break myself.

Chapter 14
Temperature

One of the ways to relax me physically is to put my body in a very specific position and to try and keep me cool, whether by cooling the room down or putting an ice pack behind me. When you have nerve damage, or some neurological issue, for the most part, your body overheats. For me, I always feel cold on the inside, but my body most of the time is always warm or gets too warm.

I am very stubborn. I know I am not supposed to be in extreme heat, but since the temperature regulation is off, I feel better when I'm in the heat. People didn't understand this, and they became uncomfortable when the room temperature was set for my comfort. Everyone around me would get so frustrated that they would take their anger out on me. No one had a solution. My physical therapist and my occupational therapist did not approve of my position. My nurse knew I was in pain, but she was confused about what to do.

Chapter 15
Fourth Grade

During these years, school was getting a little bit easier, depending on the teacher and the aide I had for each grade. I have to say that one of the worst school years was fourth grade. I did not like the teacher, but, more important, I had two major surgeries that year to ease my spasms. My body, especially my nervous system, takes a while to heal. Slow healing is difficult because I can be very impatient. This is one quality that my dad, my brother, and I all share. *Hey, we're Italian; you have to love us.*

That year was a major struggle. I had a teacher and an aide who did not understand my situation at all. I am a slow worker, depending on what I have to do. Everything that is easier for most people is harder, more painful, and more complex for a patient with a spinal cord injury, or any disability. I would get yelled at for incomplete work when I was tired from having two surgeries in one year.

If you had asked me when I was having those surgeries if I thought they were helping, I would have said "no." Now, many years later, I can feel the impact. *How's that for slow healing?* But while my body healed over time from the surgery, my heart and mind remained somewhat injured from being yelled at and shamed that year and when I first started school.

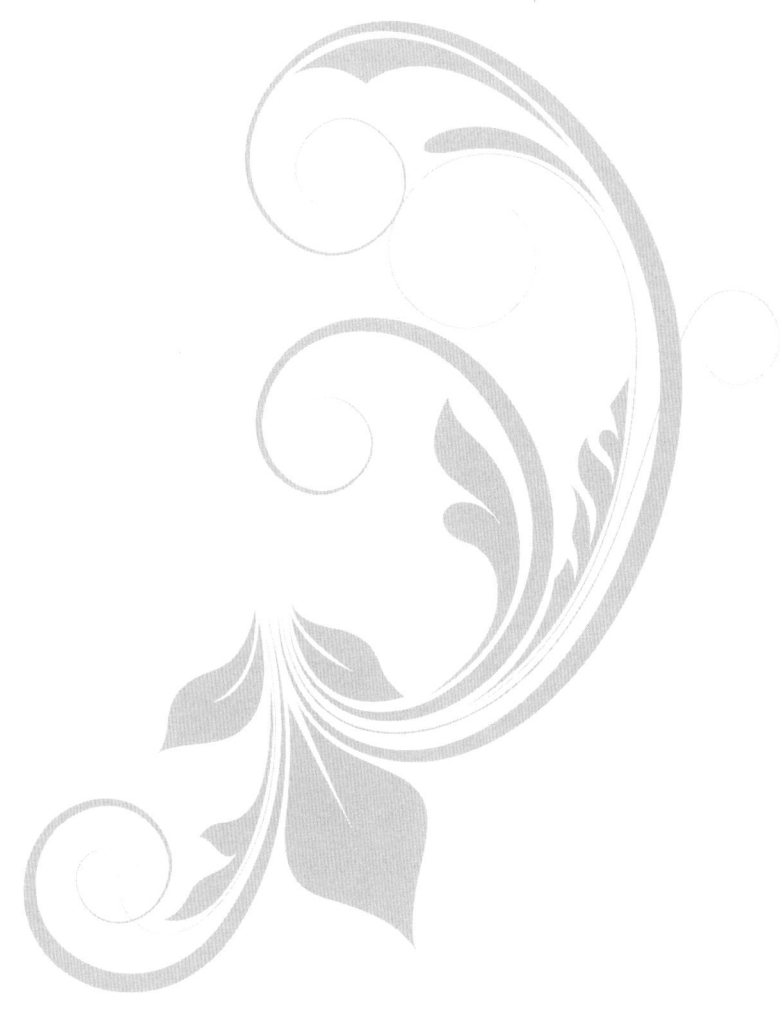

Chapter 16
Camp Friends

When I was five to twelve years old, I went to a camp run by Bergen County Special Services. I made some good friends there, including Amanda, Rachel, and Jonah. Amanda deals with challenges even greater than mine. She can't speak, and she can only move one finger. We connected. I could sense some of her feelings. In fact, I could express them for her. In some instances, this was very important: when her line would come out and no one noticed, I would immediately respond and alert someone. This is when I began to develop my passion for speaking for those who can't speak.

At that time, Rachel and Jonah were still so isolated by their disabilities that they were less sociable than I was. I've kept in touch with them and have been able to sense their progress. How sociable are they now? They're dating. This supports my belief that everyone is always growing. Give people a little time, and they may surprise you. One of the sayings that I like is "don't judge a book by its cover." What you might think a person is feeling, thinking, and going through may not be what is really going on. That is another reason that it makes me happy that we are all growing; some just take longer than others.

Chapter 17
Mother

At home, my mom and I were clashing. There was a lot on each of our plates. Although I didn't recognize this at the time, she was performing amazingly well given all that she was facing. At the time she had a quadriplegic daughter, a three-year-old son, and a mentally ill husband. Every time I would spasm, she would seemingly take out her frustrations on me (*like everyone else would do*). So I thought everything was my fault. Now I know better. I understand her motives and emotions much better than I did back then.

There are scars from this period deep in my soul, but my mother and I now try to get along better than any teenager and her mother that I know of. That's a good thing because I depend on her every day, not just for all the tasks that she does for me, but also for her companionship, advice, and affection. She's the best. She is my main caretaker and confidant, and even though I hate to admit it, she knows me the best. As I get older, I tend to feel guilty somewhat because she does so much for me. I respect her in my own way, and I can't imagine my life without her. I feel like I owe her, but I know that I don't. I know that she loves me, but I wish I could make it up to her some way. She still is amazing, but as she gets older, I tend to worry about her more. In order to not let this get to me, I just have to focus on the positive. Alhamdulillah, we are doing fine. I am incredibly grateful for her. *Even if it's hard to admit.*

Chapter 18
Father

So far, you have read a few things about my father: he stayed by my side the whole time I was in both the hospital and rehab while my mother was recovering; he advocated strongly for my being able to attend school; he is a primary source of my love of music. You may have noticed that I mentioned that he wasn't around some of the time. That's because he was battling with his own emotional and mental challenges, which had been aggravated by the accident and its aftermath.

There's more to him than that. Among other things, he is the source of my Italian identity. I feel Italian in my heart and in my bones. I deeply regret that my grandfather from my father's side was so busy tending his businesses that he wasn't much of a family man and didn't pass along much of the Italian culture and traditions to my father's generation and to mine. Despite that, I look Italian. I sound Italian. To a large extent, I have the same temperament as my father. So does my brother Jib.

That gets us back to the issue of mental illness. I worry and wonder how much of that Jib and I may have inherited, too. For example, I know that I have "no filter" compared to many people who are more socially refined. What I don't know is whether this relates to how my father, in some of his moods, can seem completely without filters. Once when Daddy and I were at an audition with a lot of young actresses, as the hopefuls streamed in and out of the inner office, Dad remarked, "They're going in and out like the Holocaust." I was embarrassed as hell.

Being "without screens" is just one of the ways that he can be different and sometimes difficult, but it gives you an idea of what he can be like. It was hard for me to get a clear picture of what was going on because some of my family transformed themselves into a protective cocoon around me, trying to protect me from my father.

I'm not sure whether mental illness is part of his core personality or whether he has some kind of illness that might change in the future. One of the times he was tested at a hospital in New Jersey, they first diagnosed him as having a worried mind and lack of sleep. At this time I did not see him from the end of eight years old until I was ten years old. I was contacting him through email and phone once in a while. I would update him on how we were doing. *I would still ask my family if it was my fault that he left.*

I always worry about what he has, and I want to know what it is. I try to convince myself that the label doesn't matter. I know to be alert to his moods. When my dad is in his psychotic mode, he can do and say some pretty hurtful things. I try so hard to not take them to heart because I know that's not my dad talking; it's his disease. I have my own theory about what he can possibly have. I feel like the accident and some things that we went through play a big part in regard to his mental instability. Or it can be hereditary. Who knows? There is no set answer right now. All I know for sure is that when he is just starting into one of his moods, I do my best to appeal to his sweeter side and keep him level.

This will probably sound like I am trying hard to make lemonade from lemons, but I think there's a silver lining for me in Dad's problems. His difficulties have forced me to think more openly and honestly about mental illness. For the most part in our society, we aren't comfortable thinking or talking about mental illness. We seem to think that we'll curse ourselves if we acknowledge that it might exist. But since I had to confront mental illness in my father, I'm ready to admit that I, too, suffer from some degree of mental illness.

Thinking about mental illness is always hard. It's even harder when the situation involves family members or people we know. My dad is, first and foremost, my dad. I love him. I feel like I can never repay him for staying by me while I was in the hospital. I have a deep, nagging sense that I may have somehow caused his problems. I feel that my brother Jib and I have some role to play in his recovery.

Are these sane thoughts to have? Are they part of a syndrome that has a name? It doesn't really matter. I still long for the days when he was just my daddy and his illness was not controlling him. I don't know how long it will take me to adjust to the way he is now.

Chapter 19
Settlement

We've all heard stories about people who won the lottery or a big lawsuit and then lost all their money by making bad investments or by being fooled by con men. Dave Mazie introduced us to someone who helped us make sure that would never happen: Wade Martin. I love Wade. He really cares about us. I don't know where we would be right now if it wasn't for Wade. He is one of my best friends, and I am so happy and blessed to have him in my life.

Wade Martin

"Of all the people I have met in my over-thirty years of helping people, Antonia is by far the most positive person I have ever met. I thought I was positive until I met her. She has shown me a lot by how determined she is to 'make lemonade from lemons.' No matter whom I'm working with, I make it a point to think of what I do not as 'a job' but as helping people. Antonia brings things to a new level. She's inspiring. I would do almost anything for her and her family.

I met Antonia and her family through their lawyer, Dave Mazie, who helped them win a settlement. Dave is aware that in most cases when people get a large settlement, 90 percent of the money is gone within three years. He brings in me and my team to help make sure that doesn't happen. Our first task is to assist in the right kind of planning so the settlement can be treated more strategically and cautiously, so it lasts longer and does more.

When I first met with Antonia and her mother, Fazila, from what they said and what I saw, it was clear that they might really benefit from being in a new town, a new house, and a new school system. That's what we set out to make happen. The first step was to find the house. Fazila was reluctant to look at houses at first; I practically had to drag her. We had the help of a realtor I knew who listened carefully to our requirements and was very selective about the properties she brought to our attention. In fact, she was so on target that Fazila's face lit up at the first house we saw — the one that Antonia's Special Needs Trust eventually bought once a suitable price was negotiated. Then I assembled a team to remodel the house in Weehawken, New Jersey, to make it work for Antonia, her brother, and Fazila.

Viewed from the street, the house still retains its old-school beauty and grace. Inside, some historic touches have been preserved, but the floor plan itself has been greatly changed to add features like wider hallways, an elevator, and a backup generator that will keep Antonia's vent working in case of a power outage. The best room in the house is probably Antonia's room on the third floor. We put in a picture window so that, from her bed, she can see Manhattan across the Hudson.

I initiated meetings with the Weehawken school system to help make them aware of Antonia's needs. Again, the team approach was key. At first, the representatives of the school system seemed uncomfortable with the prospect of accommodating Antonia's needs. After Andrew Purwin, the tech specialist we had brought onto this team for Antonia, and I explained how much Antonia could do to upgrade the school's technical capabilities with Wi-Fi, smart boards, and devices as well as how eager she was to be a member of the school, they became ready to welcome her.

When the home renovation was completed, we had a big housewarming/birthday party for Antonia. The guests included all sorts of people who had been involved, such as Kim Fulgenzi of Comerica Bank who pays all the monthly bills, as well as some people who had just heard about Antonia and wanted to meet her, including the mayor of Weehawken, the superintendent of schools, a representative of the Christopher Reeve Foundation, and my parents. I looked around the room and thought, 'It takes a village, and Antonia has a really cool village.'

Recently, I met with a young woman in Massachusetts, who became quadriplegic as the result of an accident, and her family. I was able to connect her, her mother, father, brother, and lawyer on FaceTime with Antonia and Fazila. This meant they could hear from someone who had been in almost the same position that they were in. Antonia and Fazila gave them encouragement in a way I never could. Antonia now has a new Facebook friend, and they'll probably keep in touch and maybe even meet in person some day. The whole thing was typical of the way Antonia manages to reach out and inspire others."

Chapter 20
Weehawken

I was really excited to move to the town that I currently live in. I was sad to leave the only home I ever knew, but I needed a fresh start. I came here when I was in fifth grade and graduated from high school here. For the most part, I have great memories. Like any young adult, there are good and bad parts of growing up. One of the best things that ever happened was prom. The kids took great care of me, and it's amazing to see how we are all growing up in our different ways. Another thing that was amazing, other than prom and dances, is that this town is a big supporter of the performing arts, which is so up my alley. I have been in almost every school show from fifth through twelfth grade. I have good memories when it comes to performing, especially in high school.

As we got older, it took me a while to adjust to the kids who didn't grow up with me, met me in a later grade, and didn't treat me with the same respect and care as the ones I had known when I was younger. My theory is, try to be nice to everyone and if they are true friends, they will come back to you and like you for who you are. I have met and stayed in touch with a few of the people I met here, but I am still waiting to see if they are real or not. Here at the high school is where my love for musical theater grew and became a passion . . . *and slight obsession.*

Antonia Valicenti

"In fourth grade, I was pretty excited when I heard in school that there was a new girl and her name was the same as mine, Antonia. And she's in a wheelchair. She seemed shy, so I stood up and said hi.

When I found out she was moving next door, I was happy. We became friends quickly. It was nice to have a friend right next door. Our names brought us together. Then we found we liked the same TV shows, same music, same stuff. We just connected.

Over the years, we have become more than friends . . . more like sisters. She's the closest friend I have. We tell each other everything. She knows as much about me as I know about her. She'll tell me to come over, and I'll come over and hang out.

In school, I used to have lunch with her every day at school. We would have lunch in her room. I would help her with her scripts when she was acting. I was always backstage dealing with lighting, so I was available to get stuff for her. In school, she was always moving forward. People, even teachers, can be mean sometimes. Antonia never let anybody take her down.

Now that she is out of school, she's working on her acting, going to auditions. I'm really happy for her because she is getting out there and doing what she wants to do. She's always doing something, always somewhere.

We went to ComiCon together this year. I had told her all about it last year, so this year she and her brother came along. She was dressed as Batgirl.

Antonia makes you feel that people can do whatever they want in the world. You don't have to be like everybody else. If there's something you want to do, do it. She's always wanted to be an actress, and she's going for it. It's inspiring."

Chapter 21
Performing Arts/Music

I started performing when I was in pre-K for my pre-K graduation. That was around the same time I discovered I could sing. The next year, in kindergarten, I had my first solo, and that is when it hit me that this is what I want to do. I am the first person on a ventilator who can sing. I also saw my first Broadway show when I was seven years old. So all these years I just kept growing and my love for performing just kept growing. I'm getting better at it day by day.

At Weehawken High School, I had the best theater teacher. He did not just teach me about musical theater; he taught me about how to be an actress and a singer. He is the reason that I'm so strong today in what I do. I love acting and singing, but musical theater will always be my first choice. When you are in a situation and you depend on everyone to help you, it gives you the feeling that there is nothing you can do. That is why I need the people who surround me to be positive. It feels amazing when I get the support from people in terms of performing. When I am performing, whether it's in a musical or monologue or just a song, I feel free. It's as if I'm driving my chair, whether I'm moving or not. I feel, especially when I'm on stage, that whatever I'm doing I'm inspiring those who are watching. It also gives me a sense of release, and it reminds me that there is more to me than my injury.

Brad Mehrten

"Antonia was in the musical theater program that I run at Weehawken High School for every grade from seventh through twelfth, and she was involved in every production. So I was able to see her grow and develop her skills over several years. Now that she's graduated, I'm still in touch with her. Antonia is the most positive person I have ever met in my life.

I think that one of the reasons why we have gotten along so well is that I have always been honest with her. When I first met her, I told her I needed to know what she could do. She showed me. It's amazing what she can do in that chair. Then, over the years we worked out how Antonia and her chair — I always called it her chariot — could get in and out of musical numbers. She continued to educate us along the way about what she could and could not do.

I saw her passion and how much she wanted this, and it made me think outside the box about how I could incorporate Antonia and her chair into as much as she is capable of doing. It was challenging, but it was well worth the challenge because she loved the process so much. She never missed a rehearsal if she was physically able to be there. She showed up at rehearsals that she wasn't even called for because she loved theater so much. She loved acting so much.

For those of us who have known her for a long time, her chair has, basically, disappeared because it's just part of Antonia. When younger students first met her, they didn't know how to approach her. But they would watch the students who knew her just hang out with Antonia like everybody else, and it just became a non-issue. Antonia's really funny; that's one of the reasons it became so easy for everybody.

Antonia has great acting skills, and, in the right role, she's spectacular. When we did Annie, *she played the detective. She had four separate scenes in the show. She also understands the process of mounting a production.*

She also has a deep, instinctive understanding of the camaraderie that can exist in theater. I always have a 'get-together' with the cast before we go out, before the curtain goes up. We gather around, and we really get all the energy up for the show. Before the last performance of The Music Man, *the last production during her school years, she asked if she could say something before we went on. What she said and the thanks that she gave to the cast and to me was inspiring. She spoke with absolutely heartfelt warmth and love. We were all in tears — tears of joy. And we went out and gave the performance all we had.*

Antonia can be feisty — not everybody gets to see this side of her. One of my favorite stories is we were producing Cinderella, *and we were getting ready to practice the waltz number, and Antonia called me over and said, 'Mr. B. (everyone calls me Mr. B.), I would like to be in the dance number in the second act.' 'Antonia, we already cast that, and unfortunately, you weren't at rehearsal that day.' She looked at me and said, 'I already asked Antoine if he would dance with me. He said OK.' She knew it had already been cast and that it was unlikely that she would get what she asked for. But what I liked about the situation was she was asking for what she wants.*

Antonia's strong will is part of why I believe she could realize her dream of being the first entertainer on a ventilator. Making it in show business is always a long shot; but in my experience, drive is often more important than talent. Antonia has both. If she finds the right vehicle, the right role, for her acting, I see no reason why her dream couldn't come true."

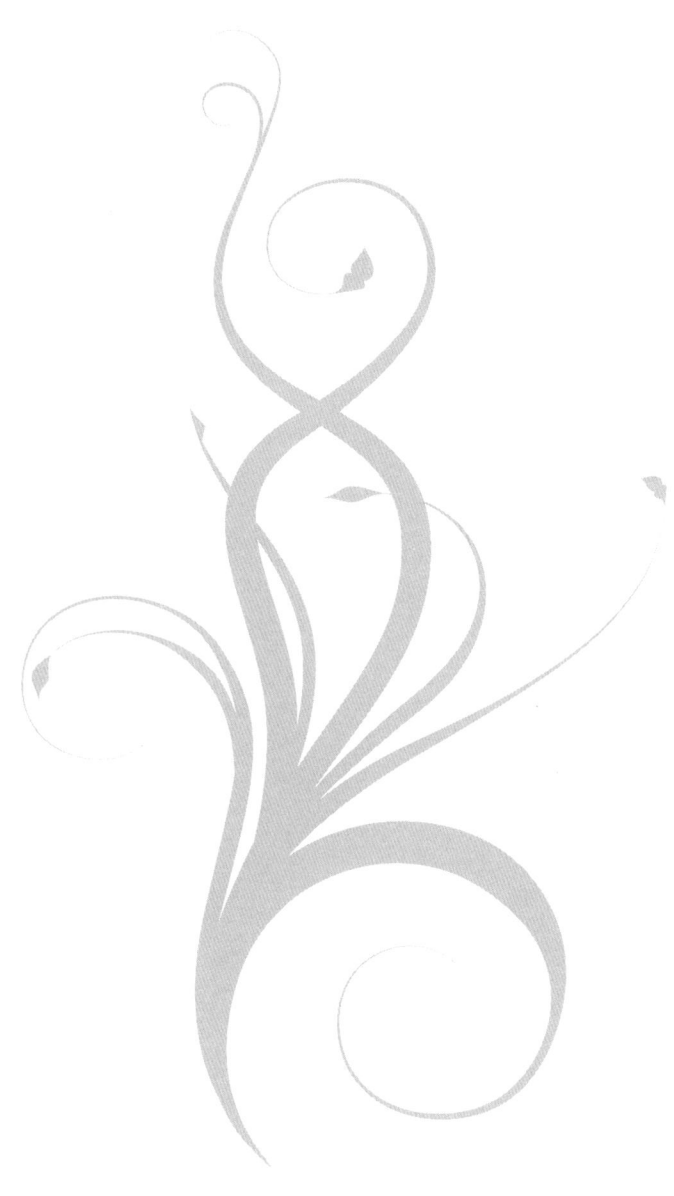

Chapter 22
Anchor

I'm the anchor of my family in all senses of the word. In the most basic sense, I am like a ship's anchor: I am pretty much stuck in one place, and my mother and brother can't get that far away from me. But there's a lot more to my being the anchor. I feel like it's my job, my responsibility, to keep the other members of my family — including my father — safe, happy, and fulfilled. When things get out of control, some of my anxiety acts up. *What can I say? I'm a control freak.*

I believe that this is a result of my injury. I have little to no control of my body. To survive, I have to be able to get the people around me to do things for me. It's frustrating needing to depend on people all the time. Like I said before, I am a control freak, and when things get out of order or things are left unaccomplished, it drives me crazy. But, I also think that part of this is just a function of my personality. My grandfather once said before and after the accident that I'm the light of my family and those who are around me. If I hadn't been injured, I might still be the anchor of my family. I like to be at the center of things. I generally have a strong idea of how things work and how things can best be organized. *I'm not shy about speaking up.* I'm not just a control freak because of the injury, although I think it plays a huge part of it, but organization runs in my family, and I wouldn't be me if I wasn't a control freak — *but ya gotta love me anyway.*

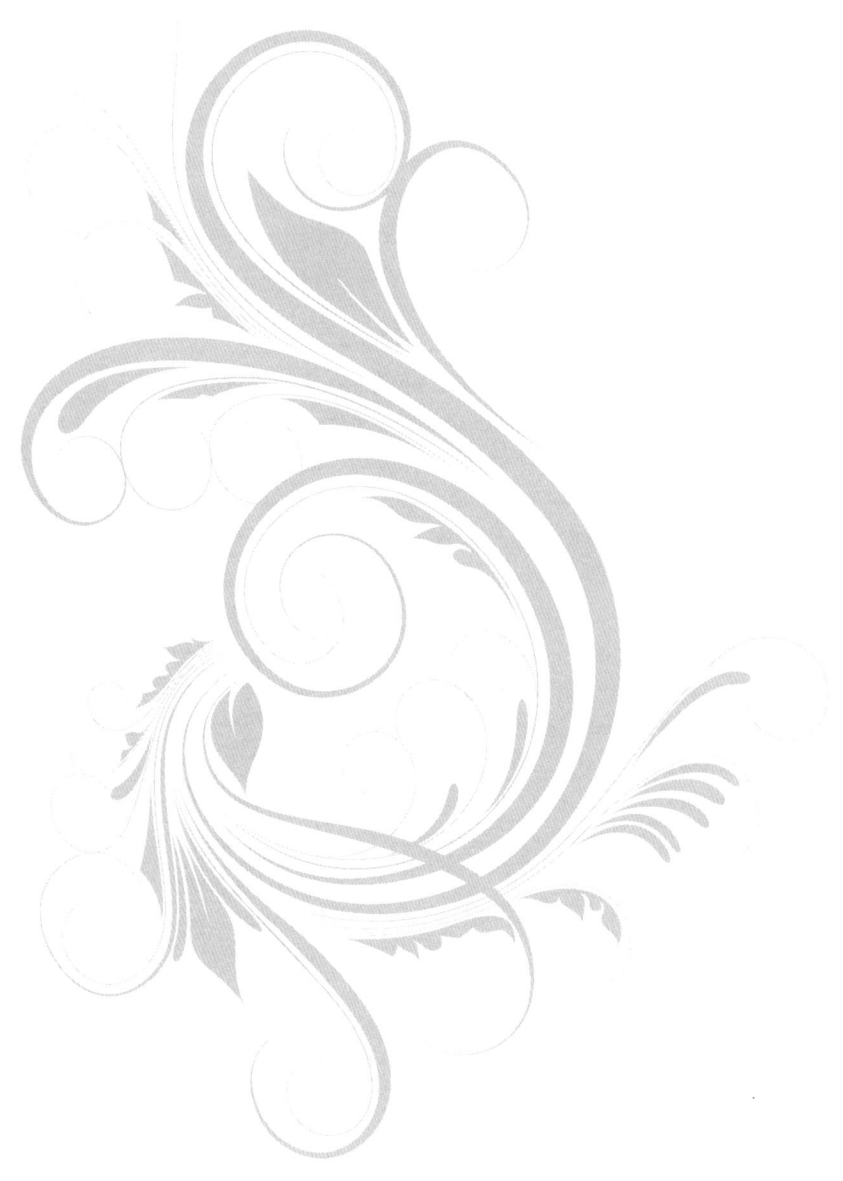

Chapter 23
Brother

I have so much emotion buried inside me because when my brother Jib was little, and still to this day, I feel he doesn't get the attention he needs because I am always taking it away one way or another. I realized this in the second grade when the guilt started coming in. I would think that my father's illness, my brother's tantrums, and my spasms were all my fault. I now know that it is not true, but I cannot always control that feeling.

When Jib was little, he said to Mommy, "Everything she does, I look up to her." When I heard that, it made me happy. I have always said to my mom (but never in front of Jib), "We may argue, but he is still my light, and I need my light." My brother and I are close, now that he is growing up and we are starting to have similar interests. I know he would do anything to help me when the time comes for it. When we were younger, whenever we had writing assignments for school, we would always write about each other.

He cares for me so much that there are times when he listens from the top of the stairs, and if he hears me crying, he'll come down and try to comfort me. He's always alert. He and my mom are the two most alert people when it comes to anything. For example, if my line comes out, he'll be the first one to put it back in, even if there's a nurse next to me. He is so fast and caring that it makes me feel guilty because he always has to worry about me.

I can sense he wants more of Mommy's attention, but he is also growing up. My mom can sense it, also. But I feel like I take it away from him. He wants a family, and I want a family, but we can't have it as much as we would like because I have Tom, Dick, and Harry all the time working with me. Only on the weekends or when we are alone can he come in and really be himself.

As he grows up and changes into a young man, he wants to be the man of the house. He wants to be my protector. I know that he has my back. He also wants to have a normal teenage life.

He's often out and about with his friends. I feel anger. I feel jealousy. I feel hurt. I feel lonely because I want to be out with my friends or I want to be out with him. *It's not easy being trapped in a body that you can't move in.* I describe this feeling as being trapped on the floor in a glass cage. But I try to be happy, and for the most part I am. I love him. I want him to have as normal a life as he can. I want him to have every opportunity that I will never have, and this goes to everybody on this planet, not just to him.

Jib

"Antonia's my sister and I love her. At times, we fight like any brother and sister would. We tease each other, as any brother and sister would. We hang out more easily and more naturally than some brothers and sisters I know of.

I'm aware of Antonia's challenges. I would be protective of her if someone or something threatened her. I can do almost all of the things she may need done, except that I haven't been trained to apply suction. But this doesn't feel like anything unusual. This is how things have always been in my life.

I think that Antonia's situation has shaped our family life. When I was little, my mom never let me do things with friends because she was like, 'I need you to be careful.' On the positive side, Antonia brings everyone in the family together. She wants everyone to show up on holidays. She wants to see them.

Antonia and I share some personality traits. We both speak plainly and directly. Neither of us likes to back down. I have no way of knowing, but I imagine that if Antonia hadn't been injured, she would be as active as I am.

The way I see it, Antonia's a normal person. She just can't move. Society doesn't always accept that. But she pushes through so she can do what she wants to do."

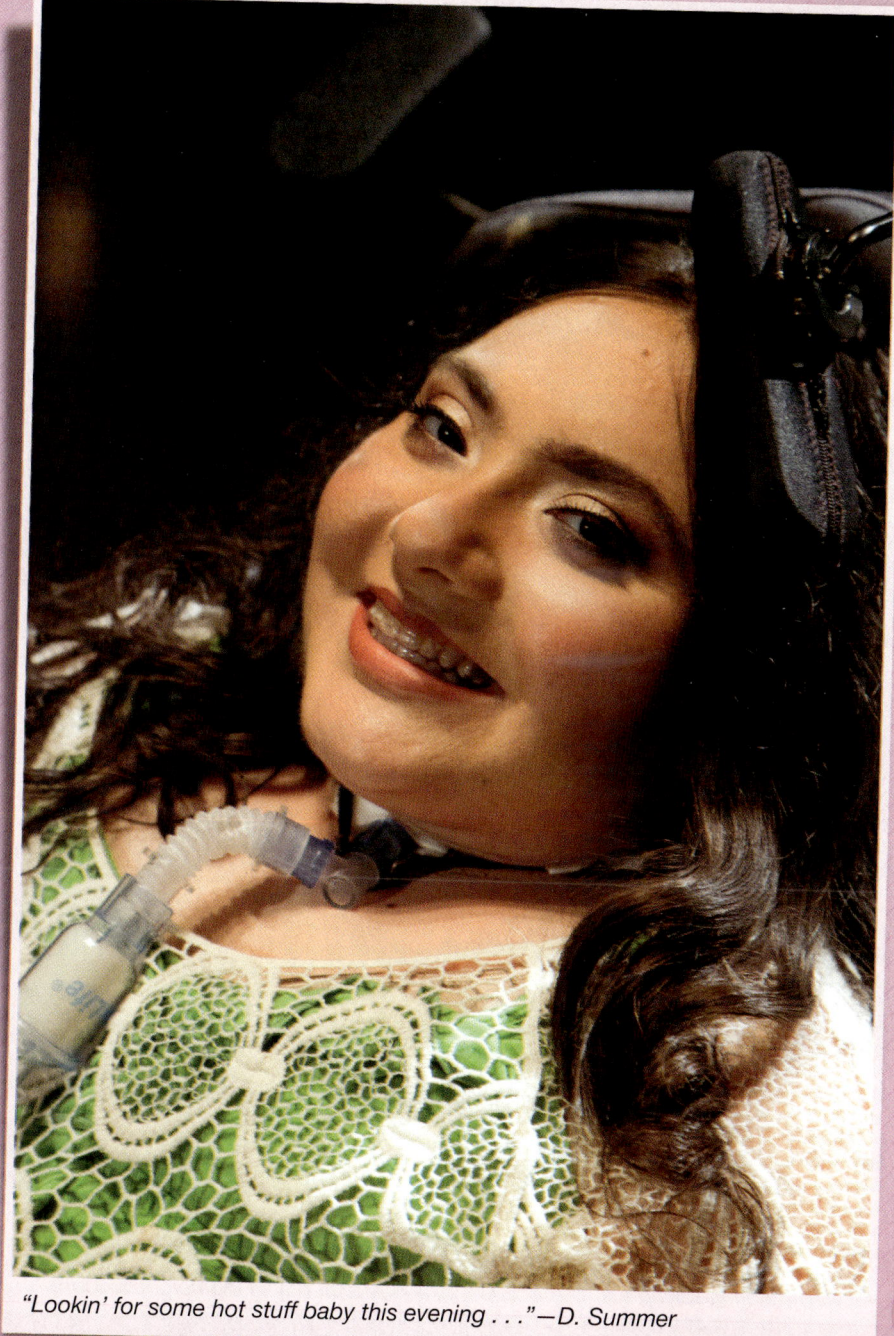

"Lookin' for some hot stuff baby this evening . . ." —D. Summer

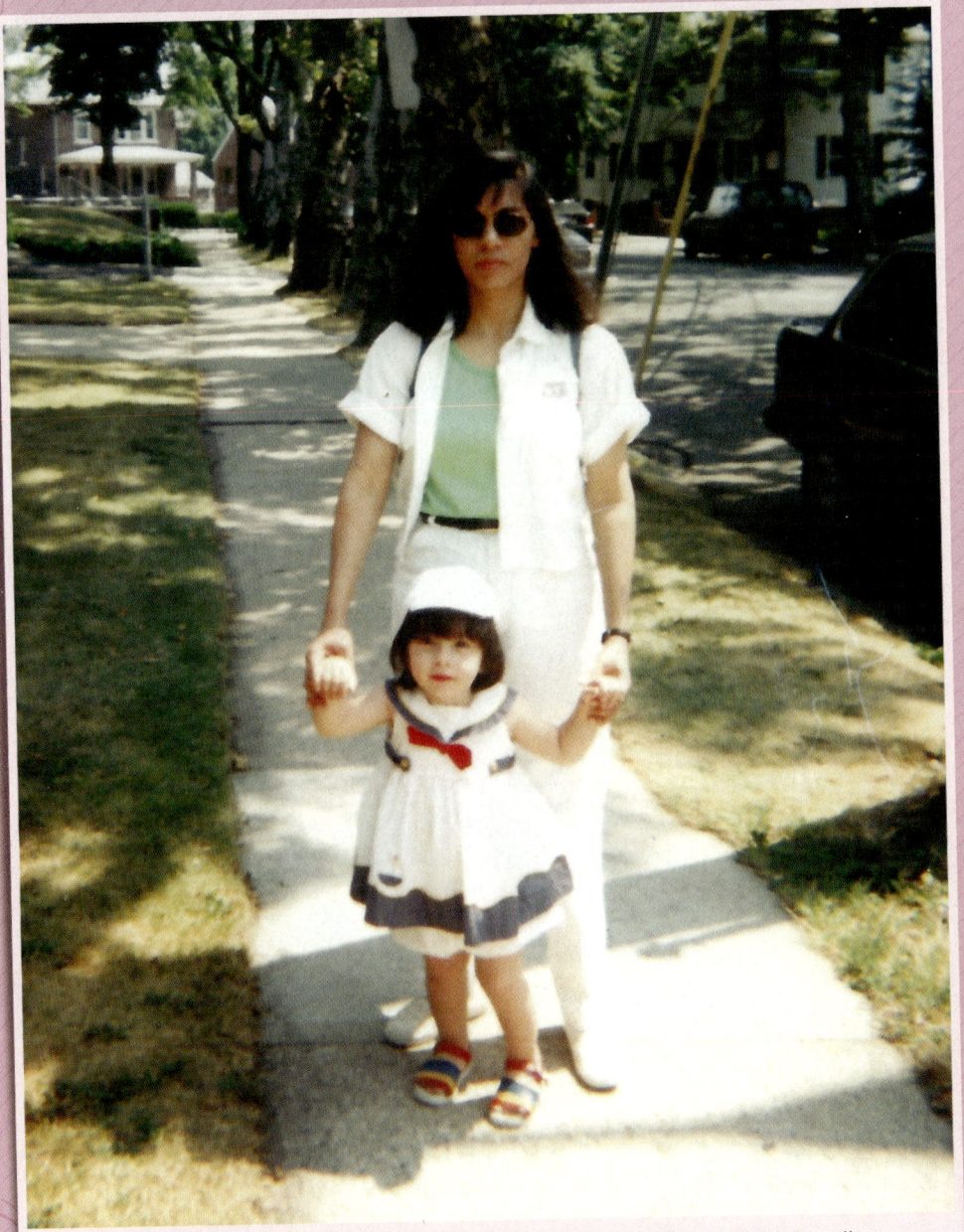

Mommy and me taking a stroll because it's a beautiful day in the neighborhood!

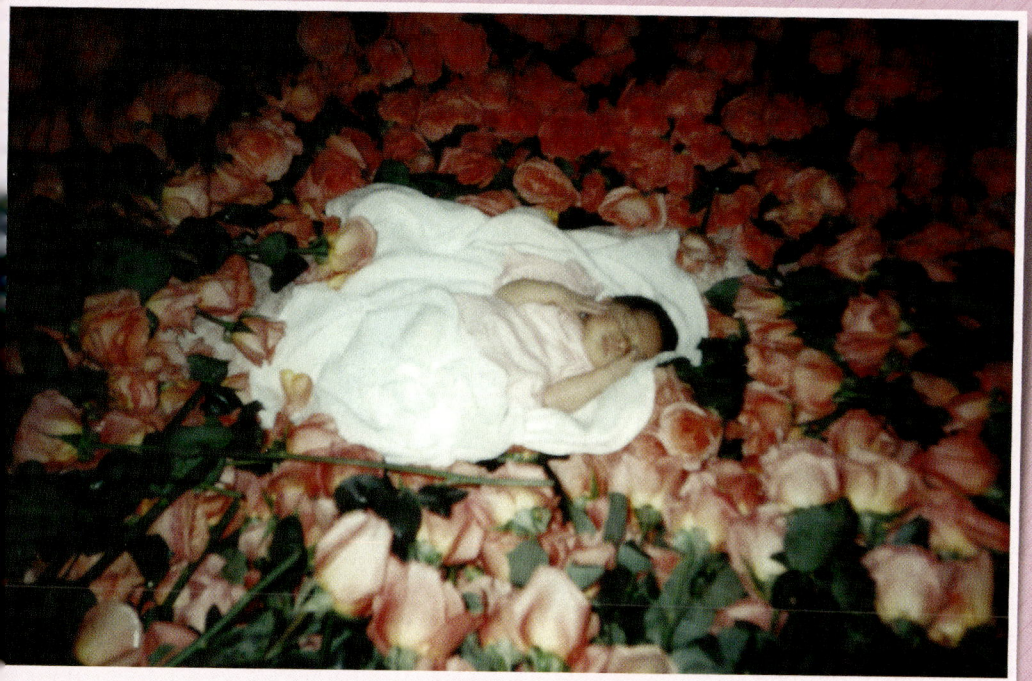
Me at two days old. The story goes that my dad bought me 1,000 roses.

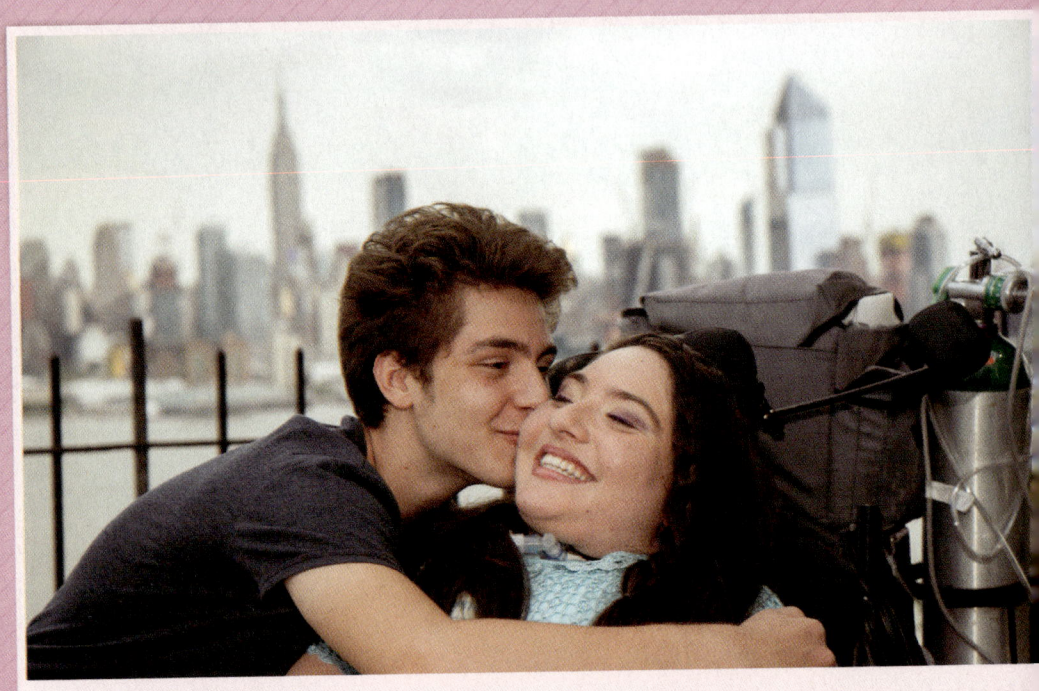

Brother/sister love!

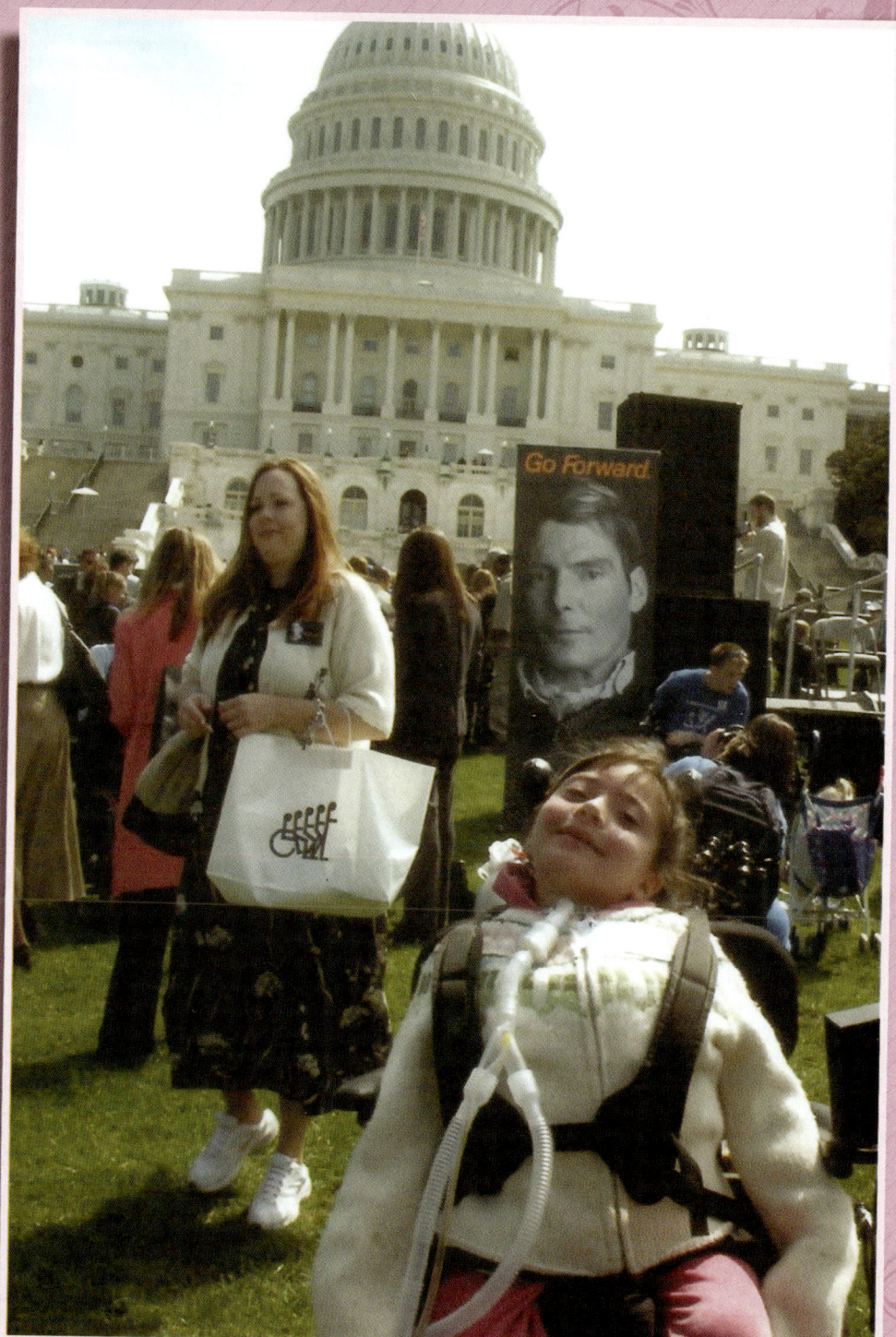
Rockin' out in DC with the Christopher Reeve Foundation, March 2005

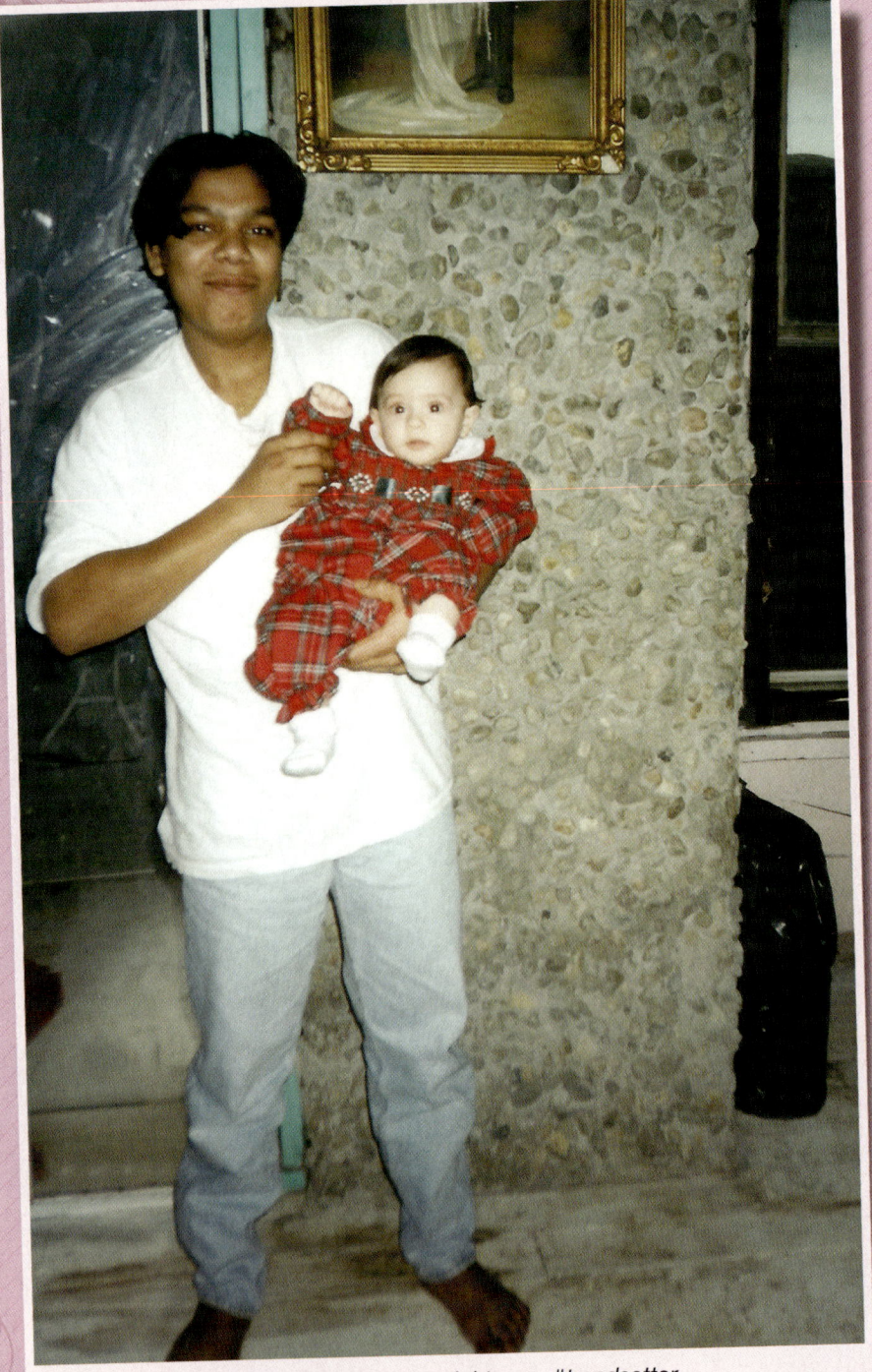
Double trouble! I think I'm fist bumping right now. #trendsetter

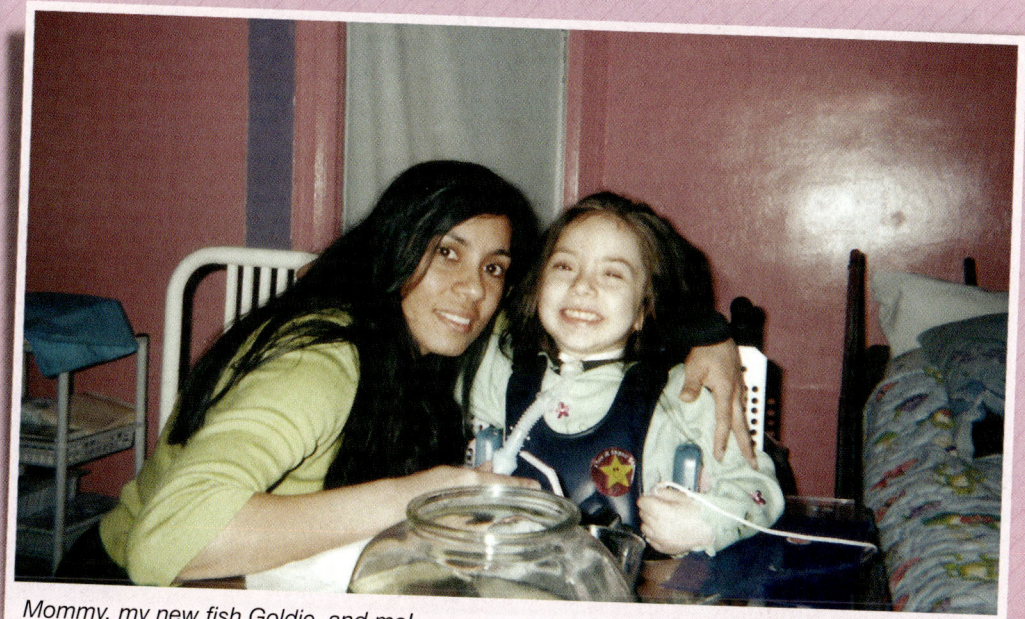
Mommy, my new fish Goldie, and me!

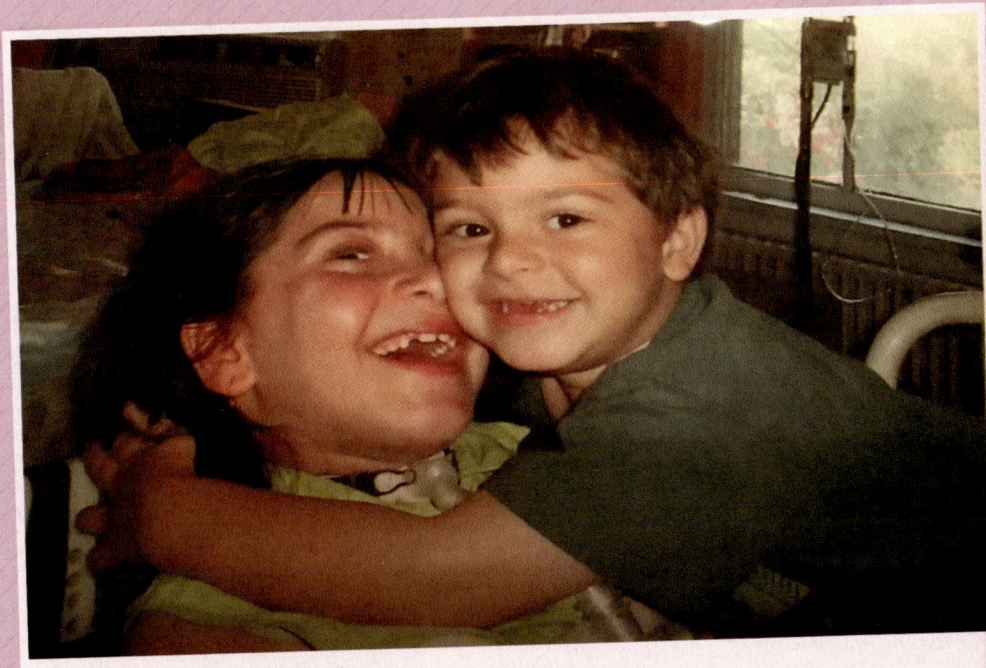
Jib and I as kids back in the day

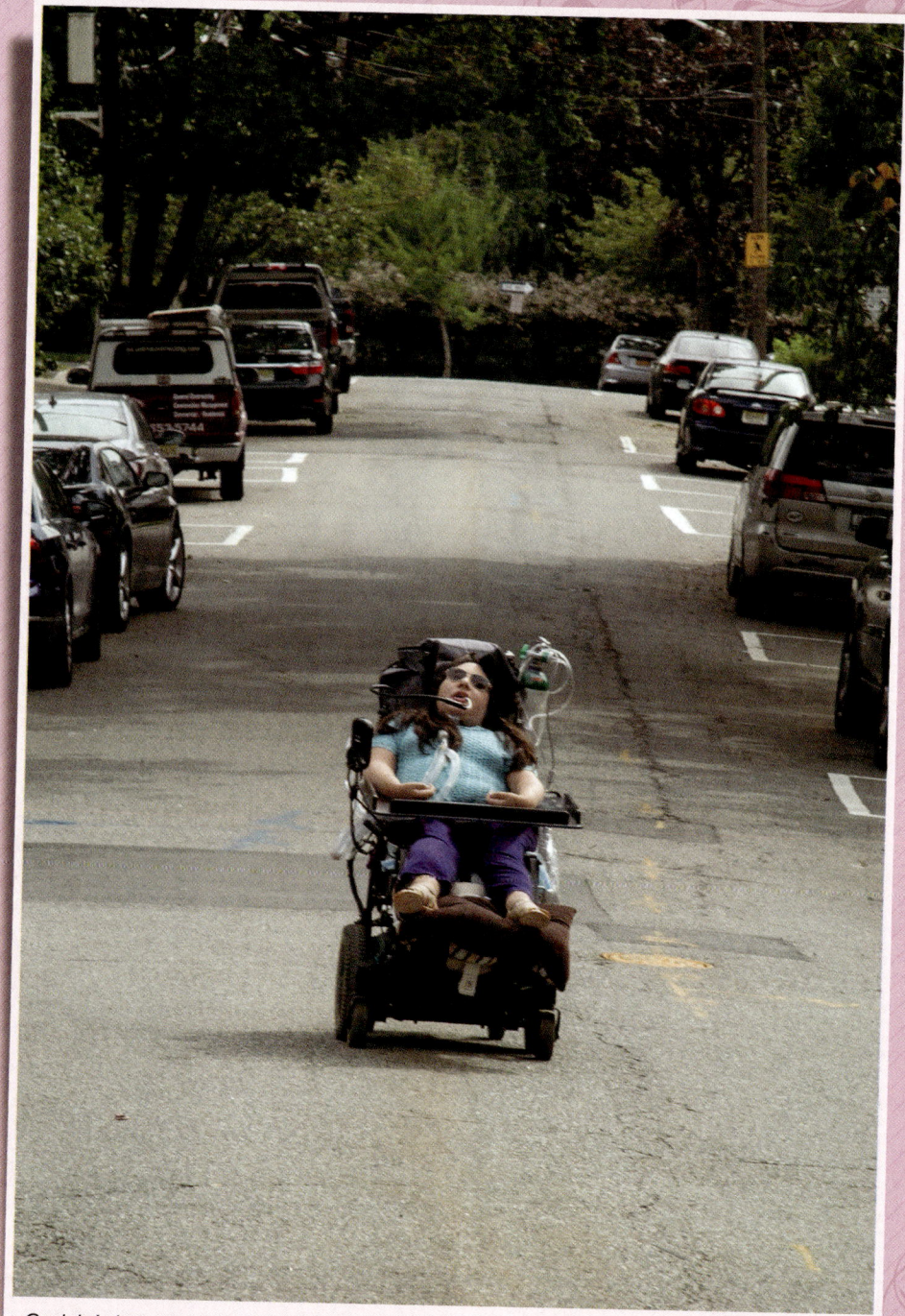

Cruisin' down the street in my six-fo

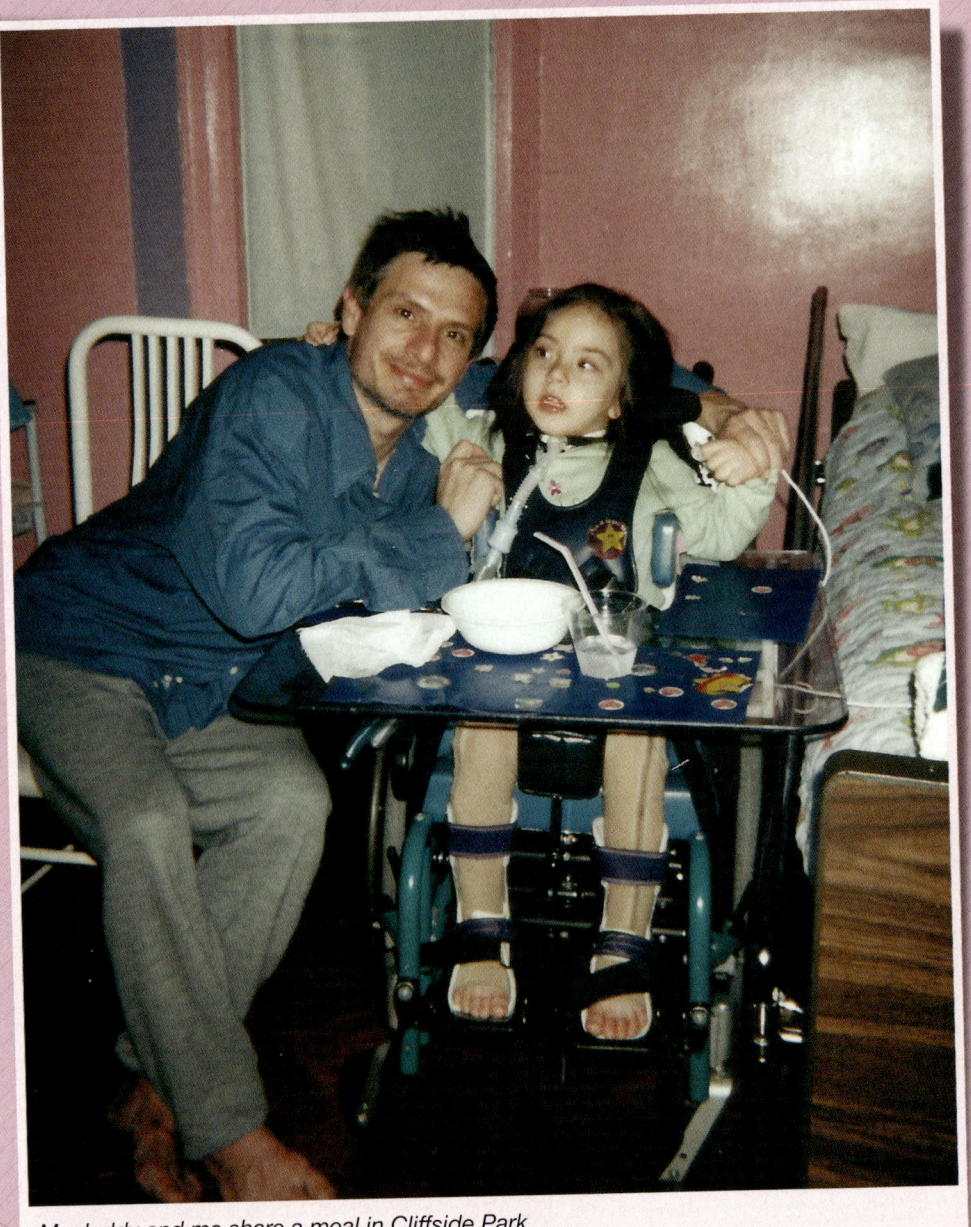
My daddy and me share a meal in Cliffside Park.

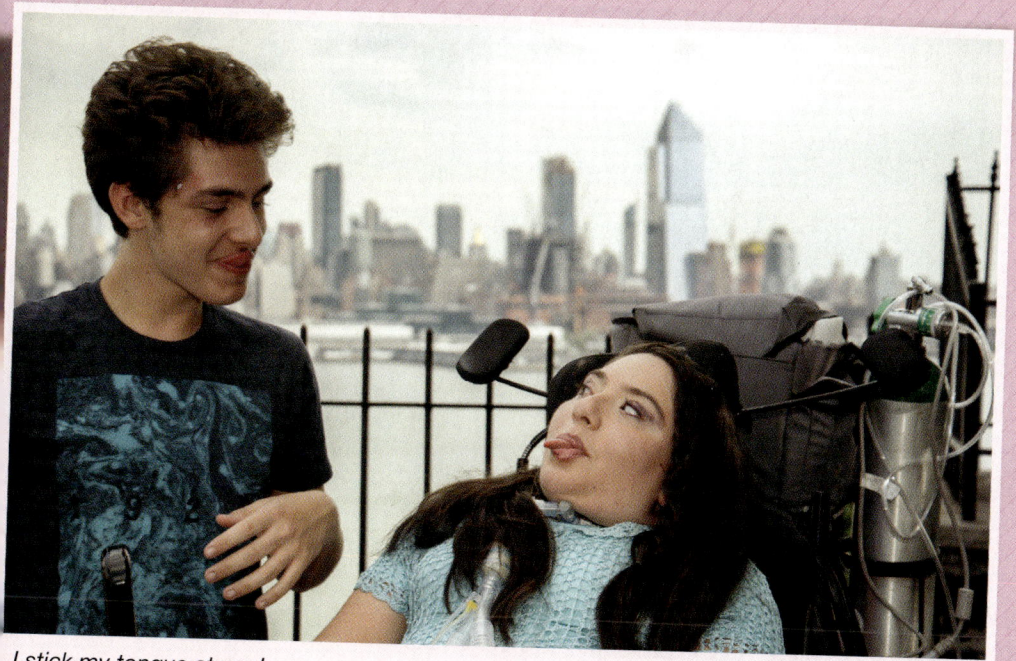
I stick my tongue at you!

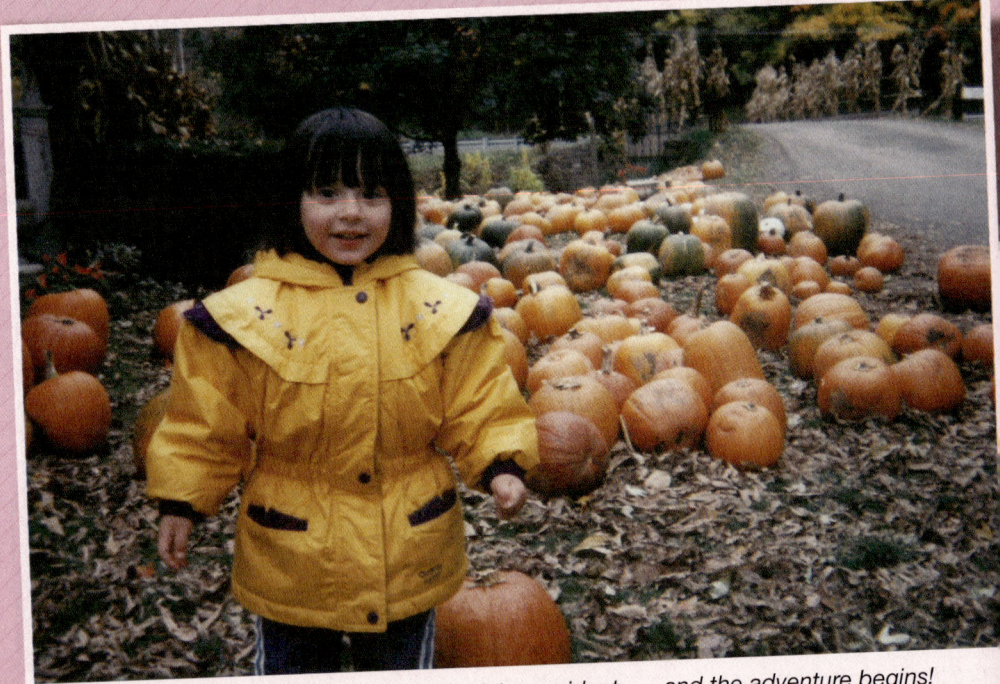
Two years old, pumpkin picking, the day of the accident . . . and the adventure begins!

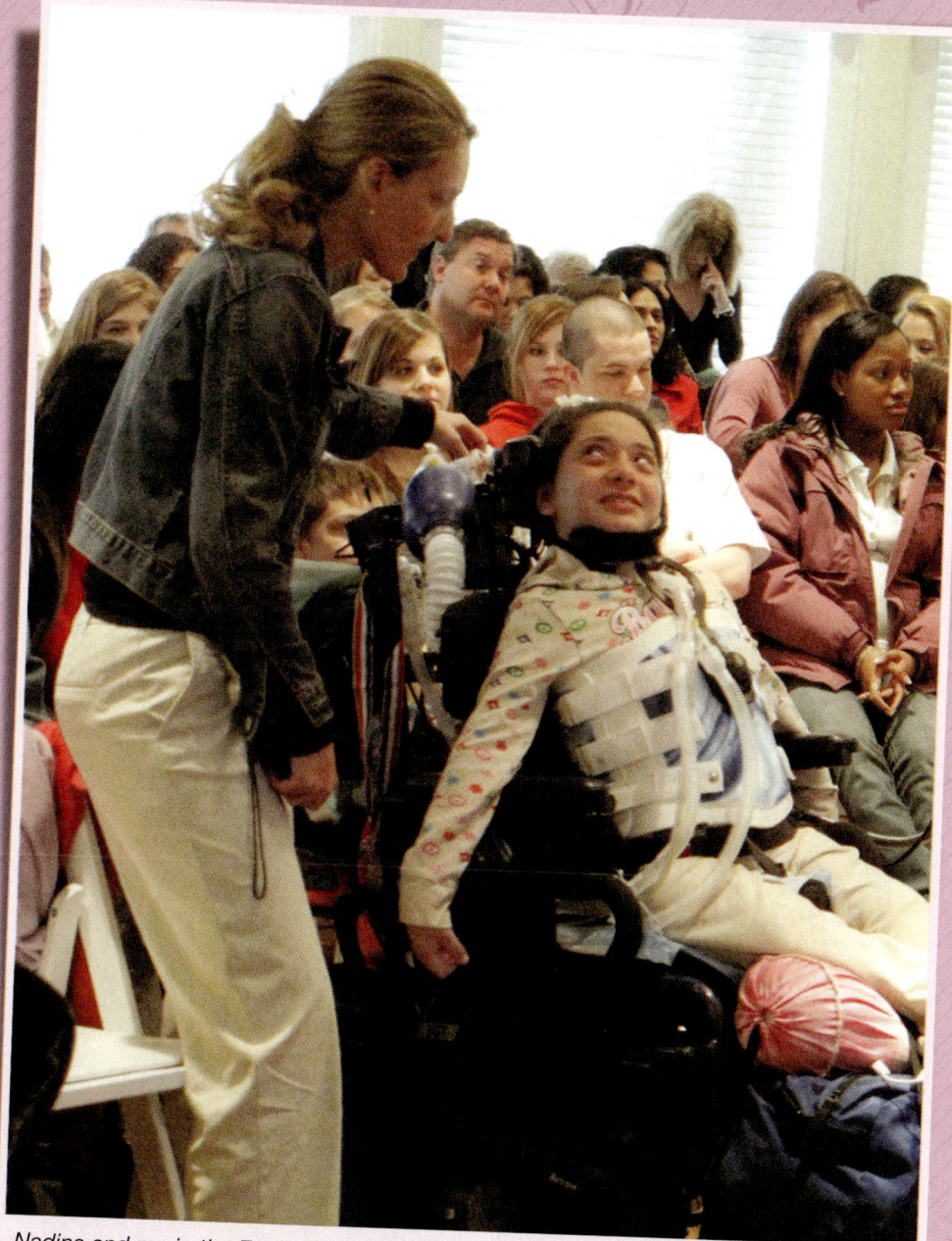
Nadine and me in the Fame Game

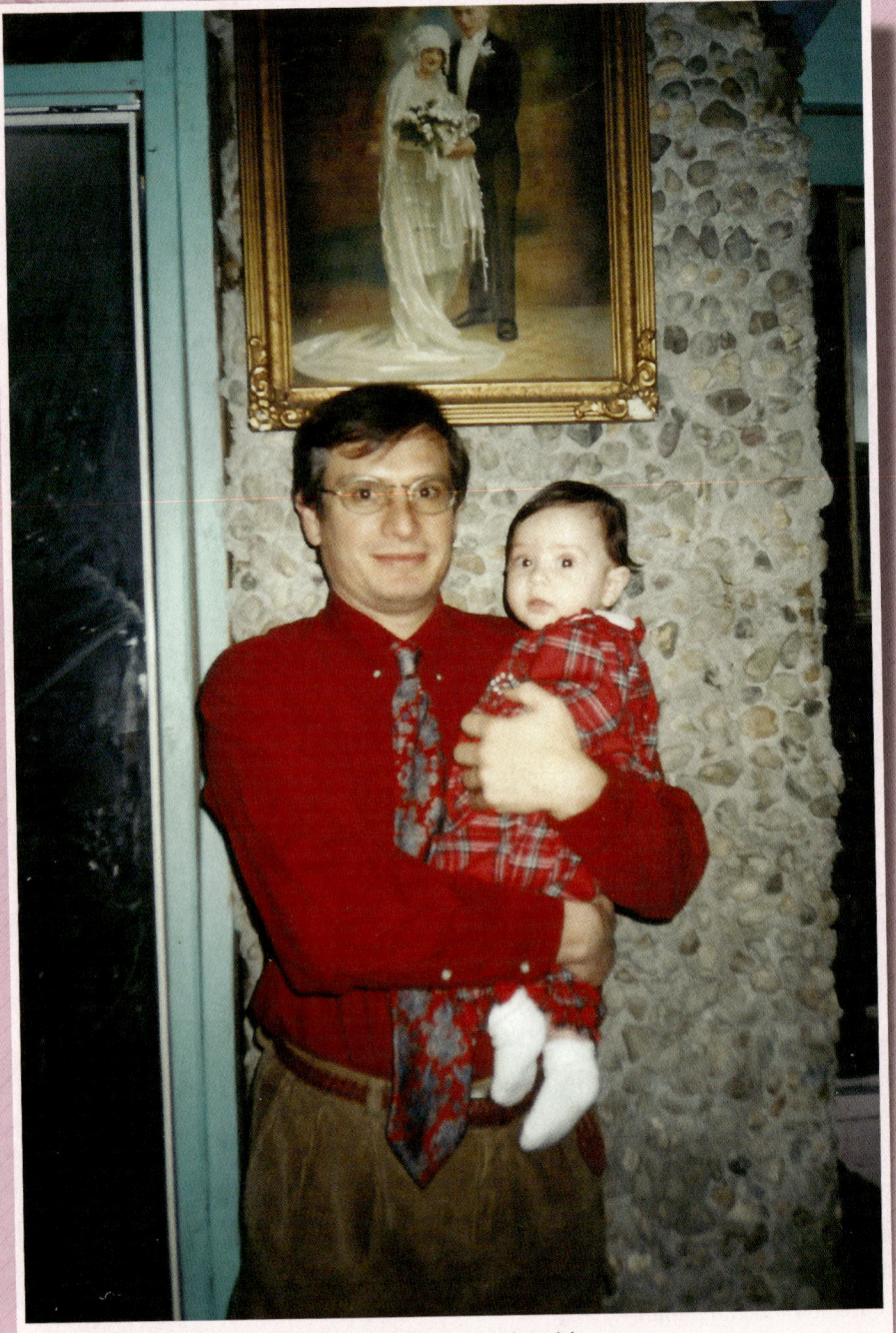
My dad and me when I was less than six months old

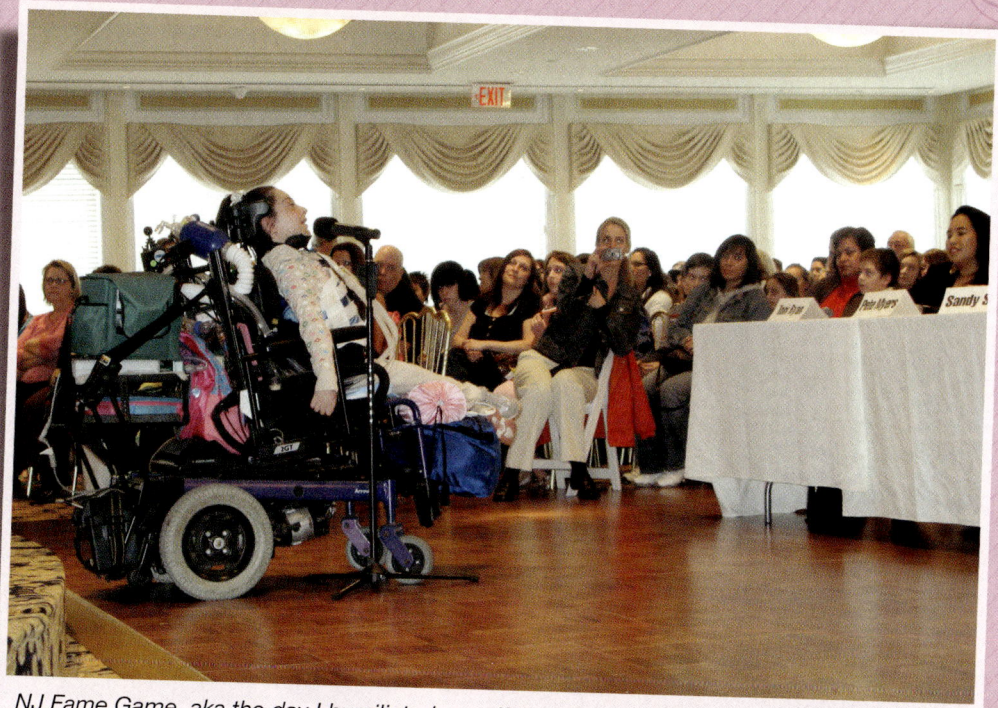

NJ Fame Game, aka the day I humiliated myself in the best possible way, April 2008. Everyone has to start somewhere!

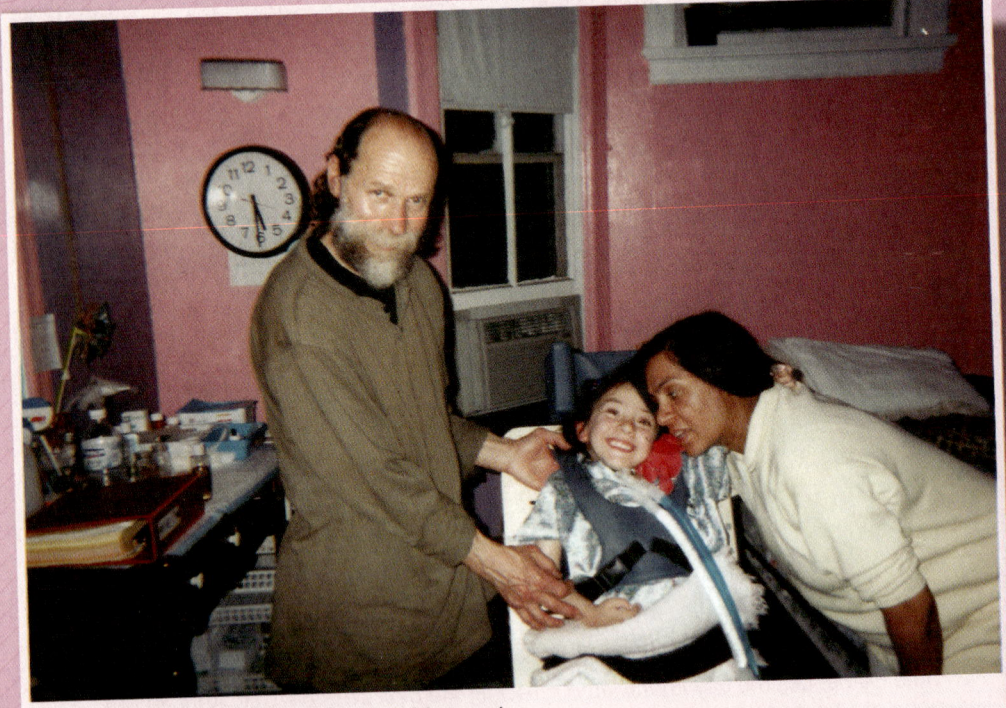

Me at five years old, with Alex, my chiropractor

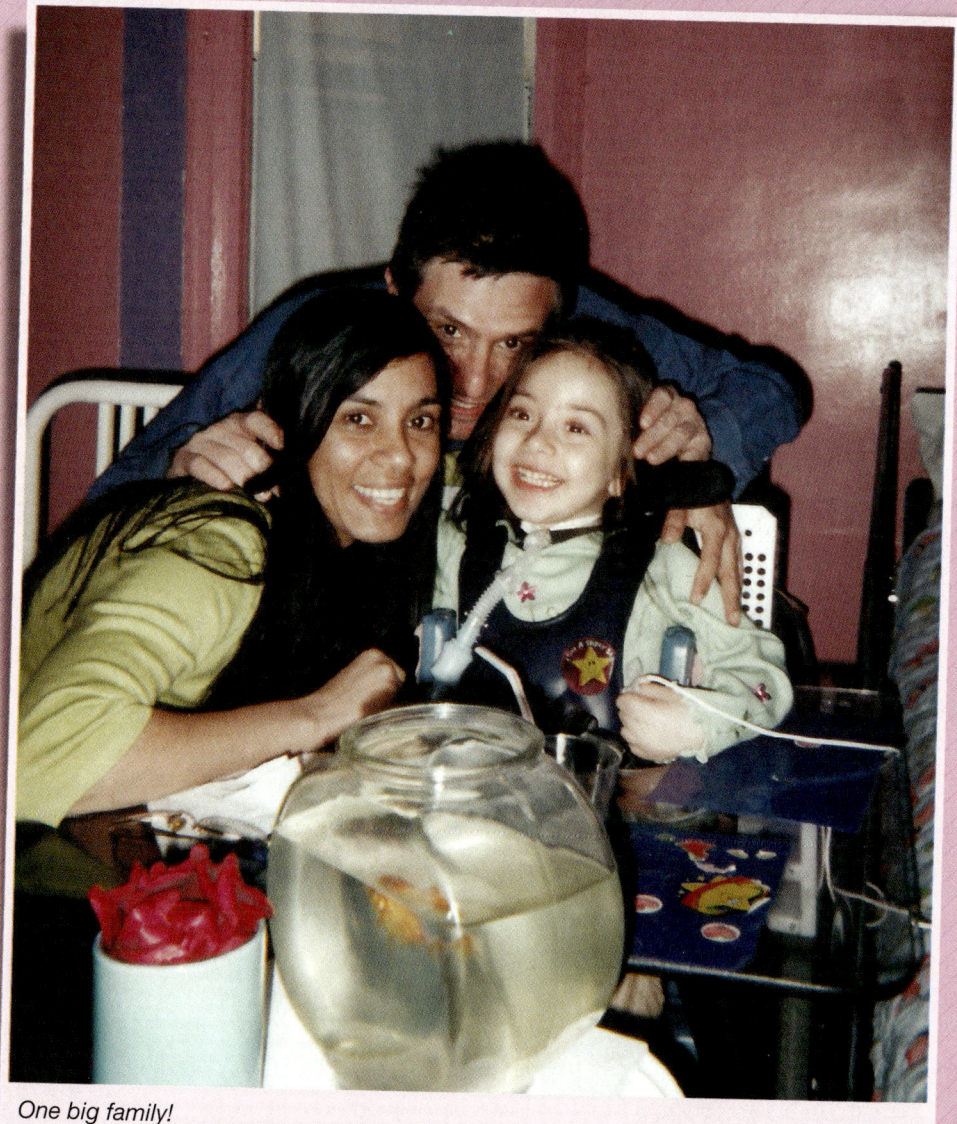
One big family!

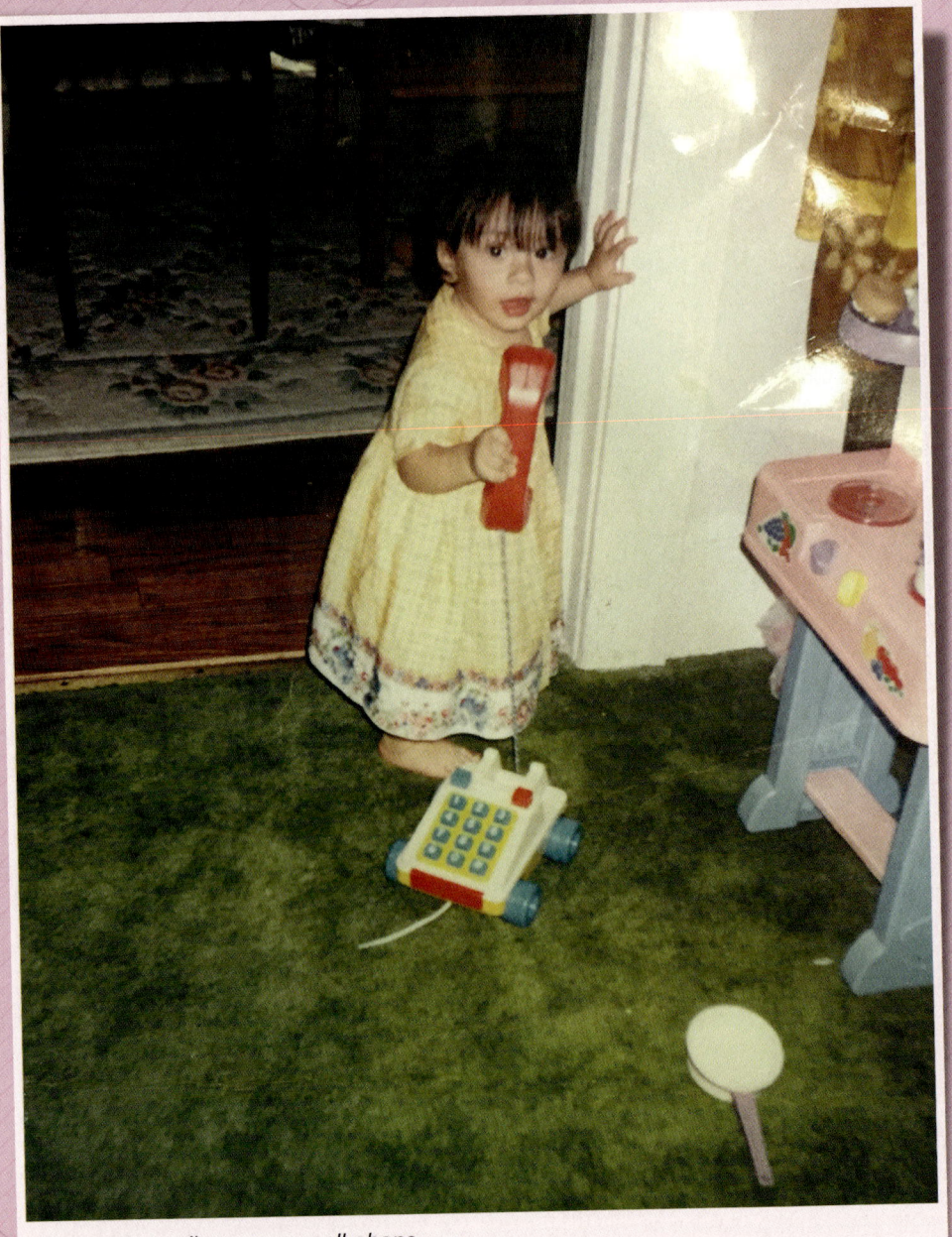

You used to call me on my cell phone.

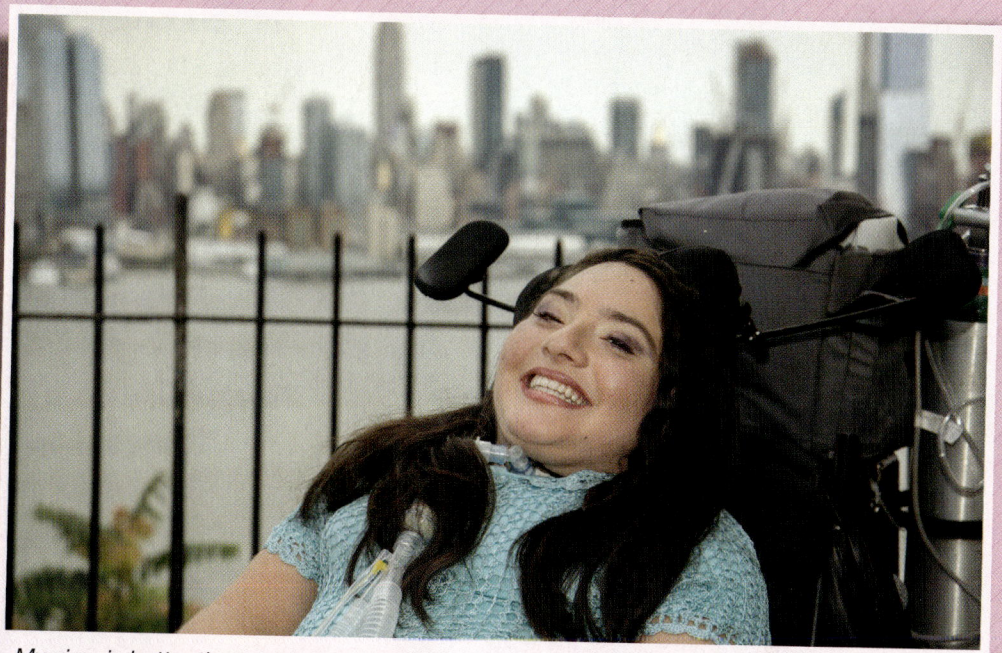
My view is better than yours muahaha :-)

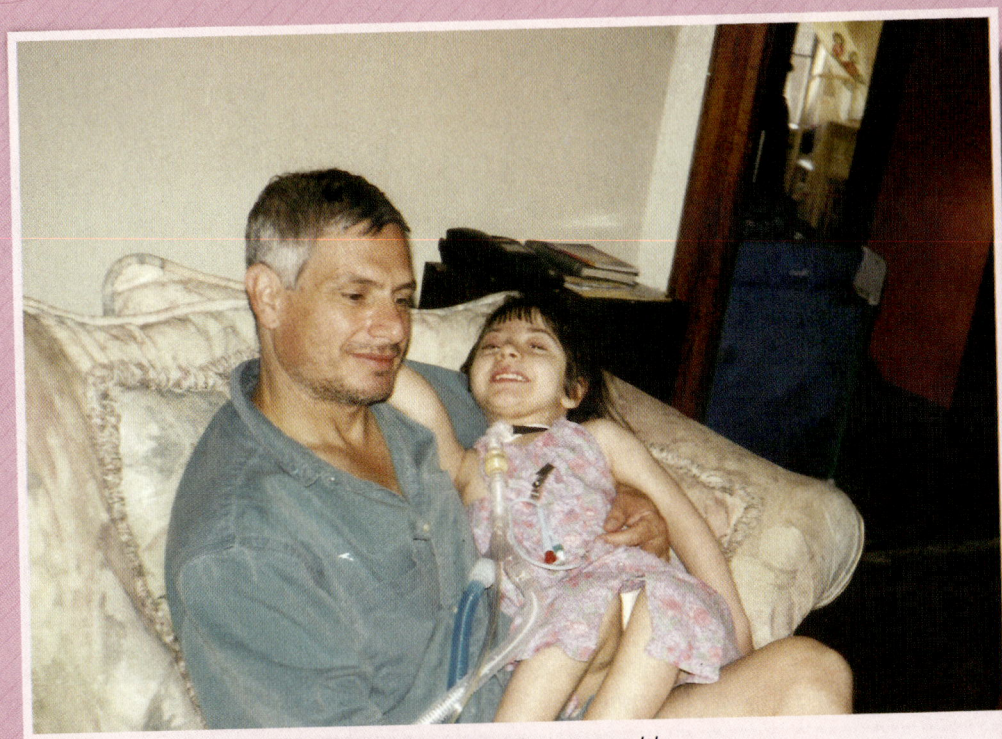
Daddy and me kickin' it . . . when I was about four years old

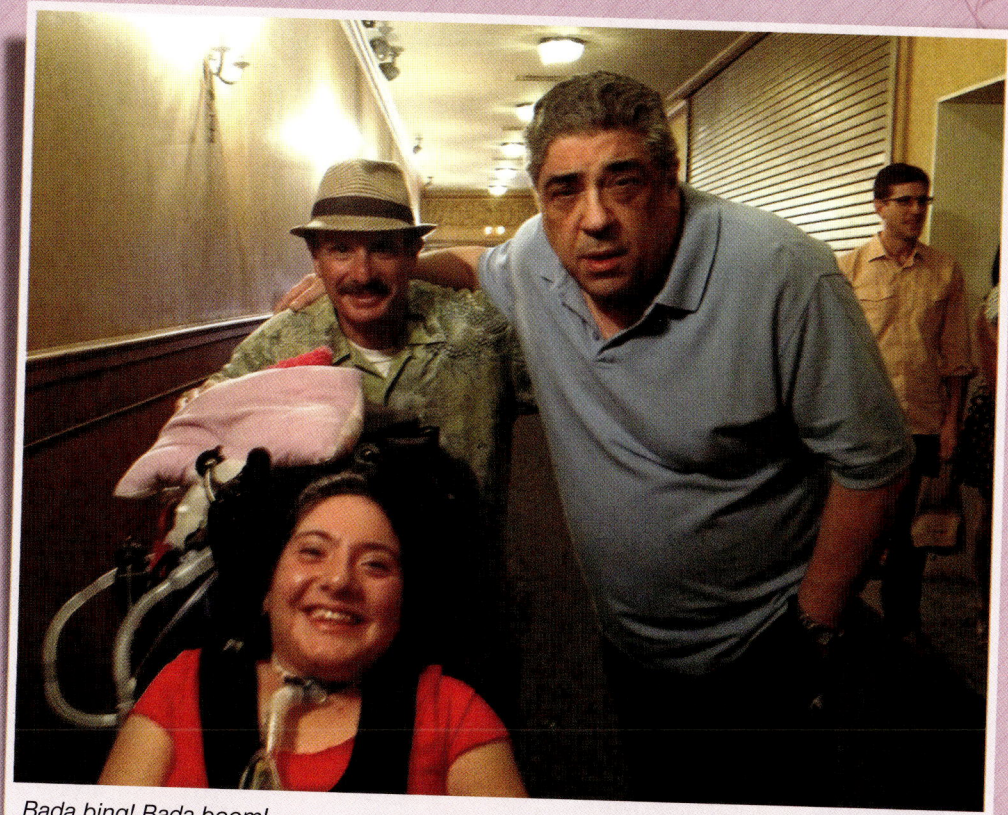
Bada bing! Bada boom!

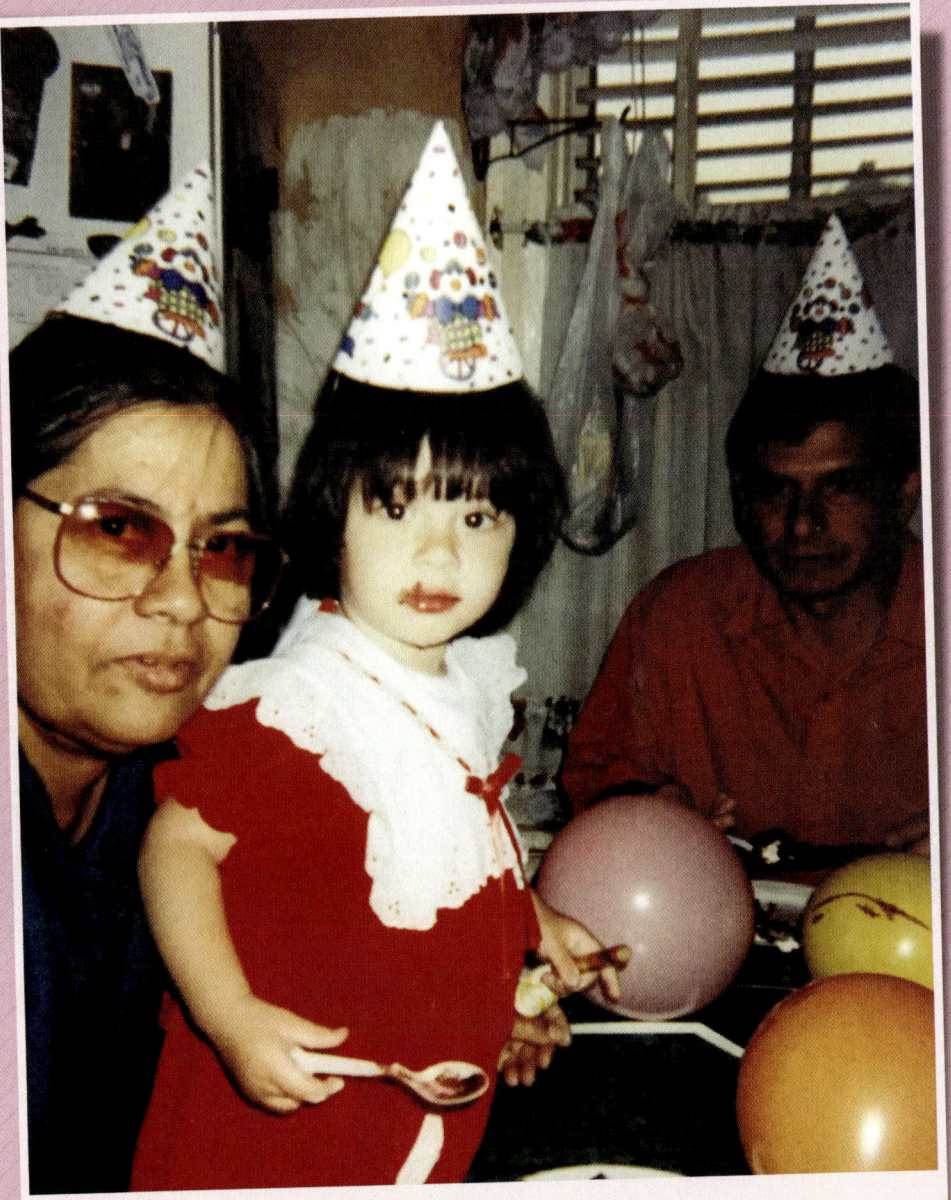

Daddy, Grandma, and me. I LOVE chocolate.

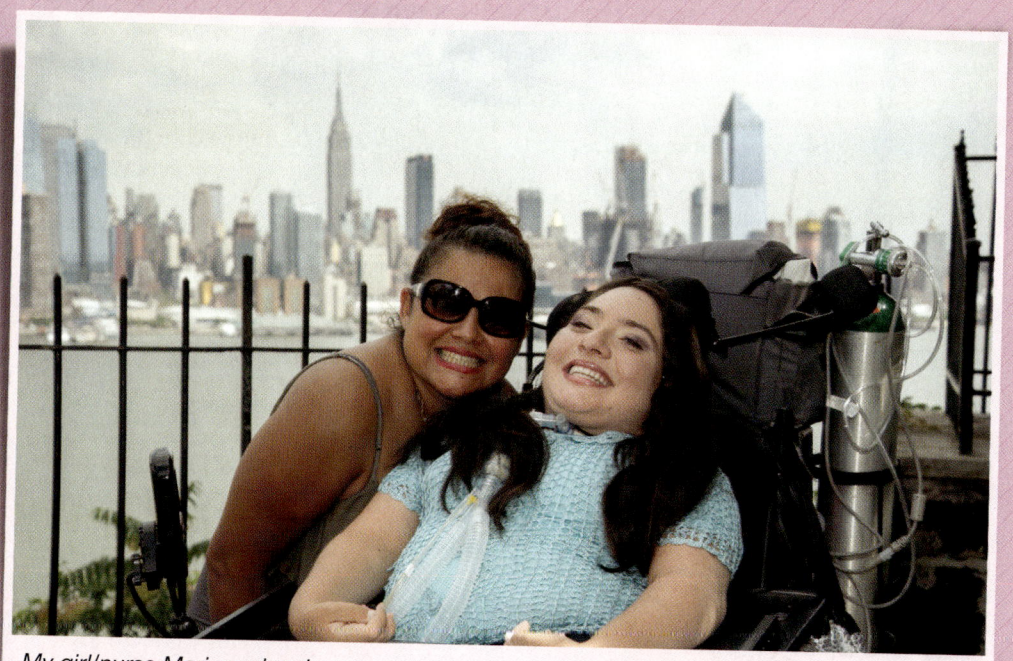
My girl/nurse Maria and me!

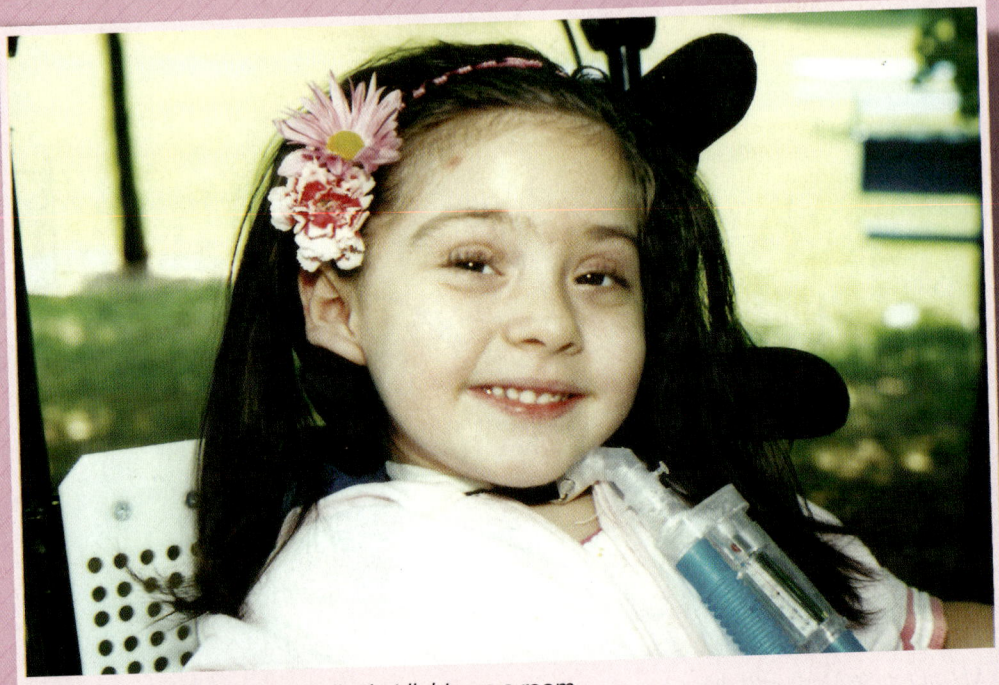
Me picture perfect with a smile that lights up a room

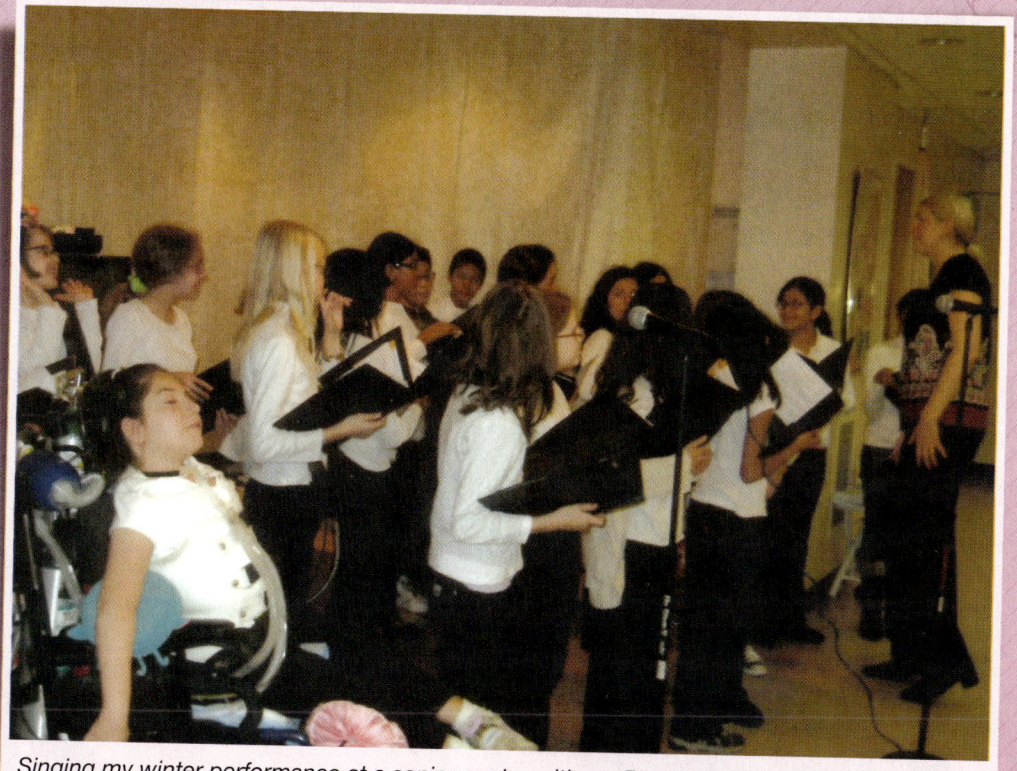
Singing my winter performance at a senior center with my Roosevelt Elementary Choir

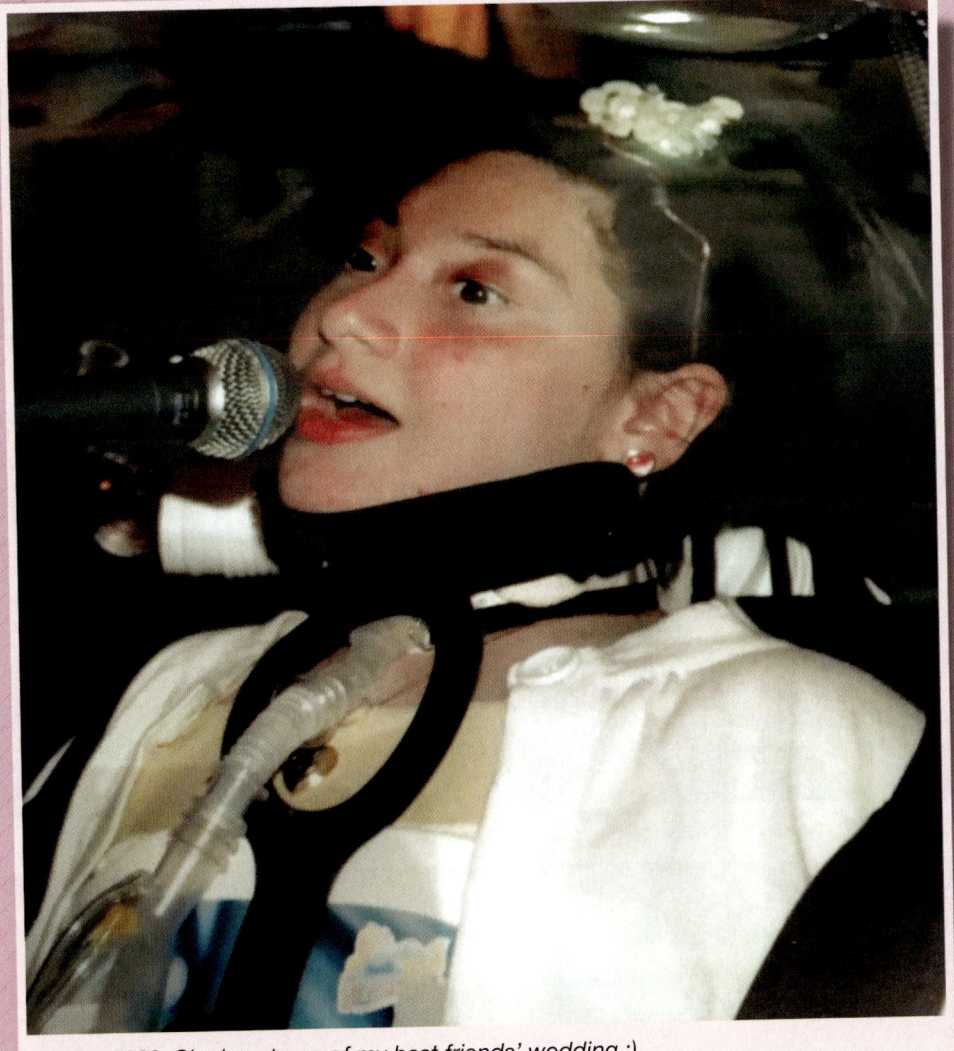

Spring 2008. Singing at one of my best friends' wedding :)

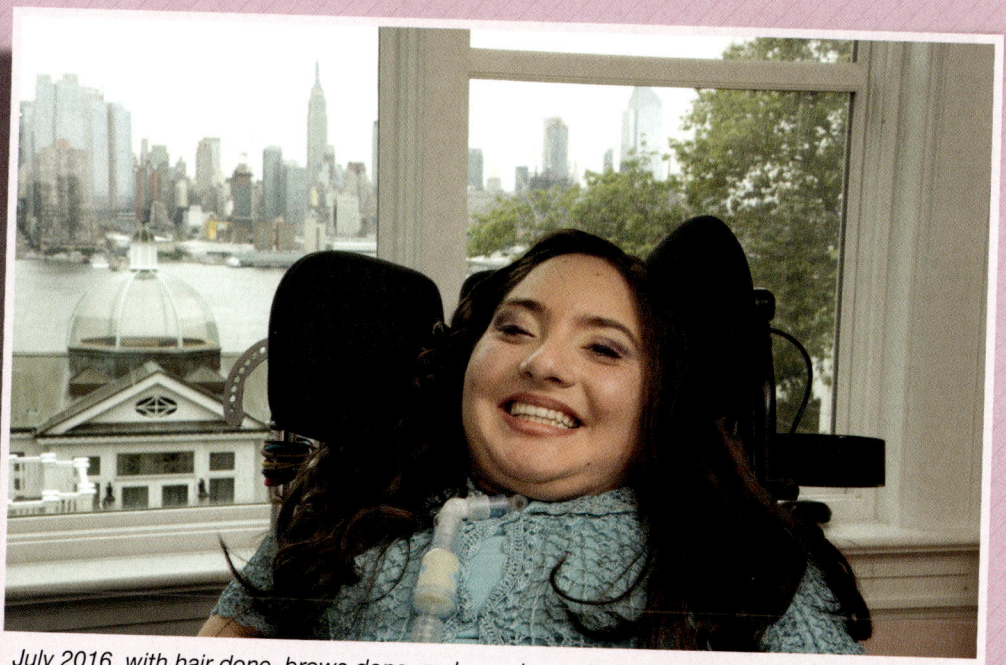
July 2016, with hair done, brows done, makeup done—lookin' hottt!!!

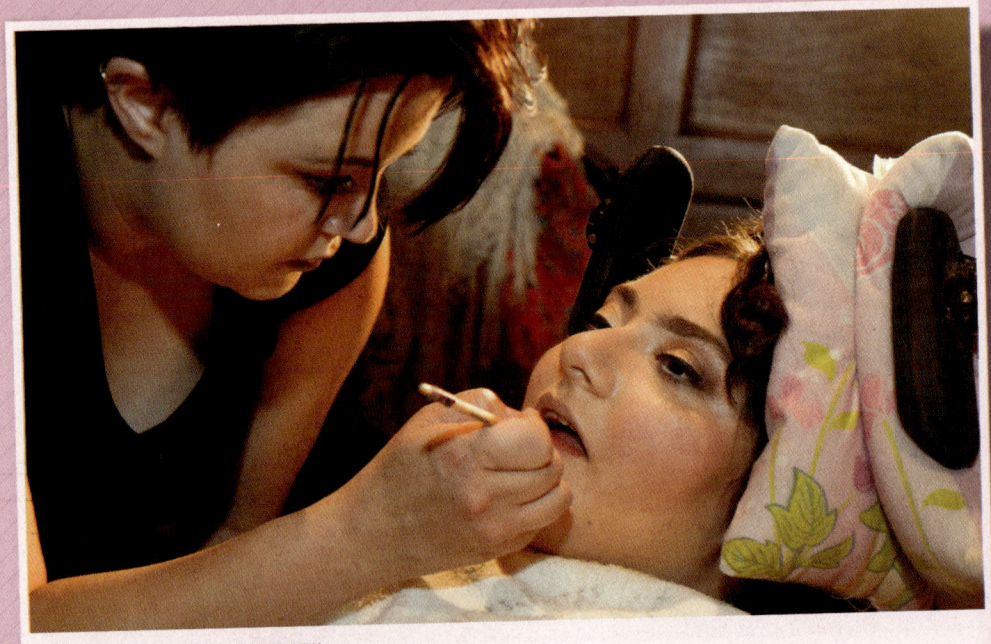

July 2016, MAKEUP TIME!!

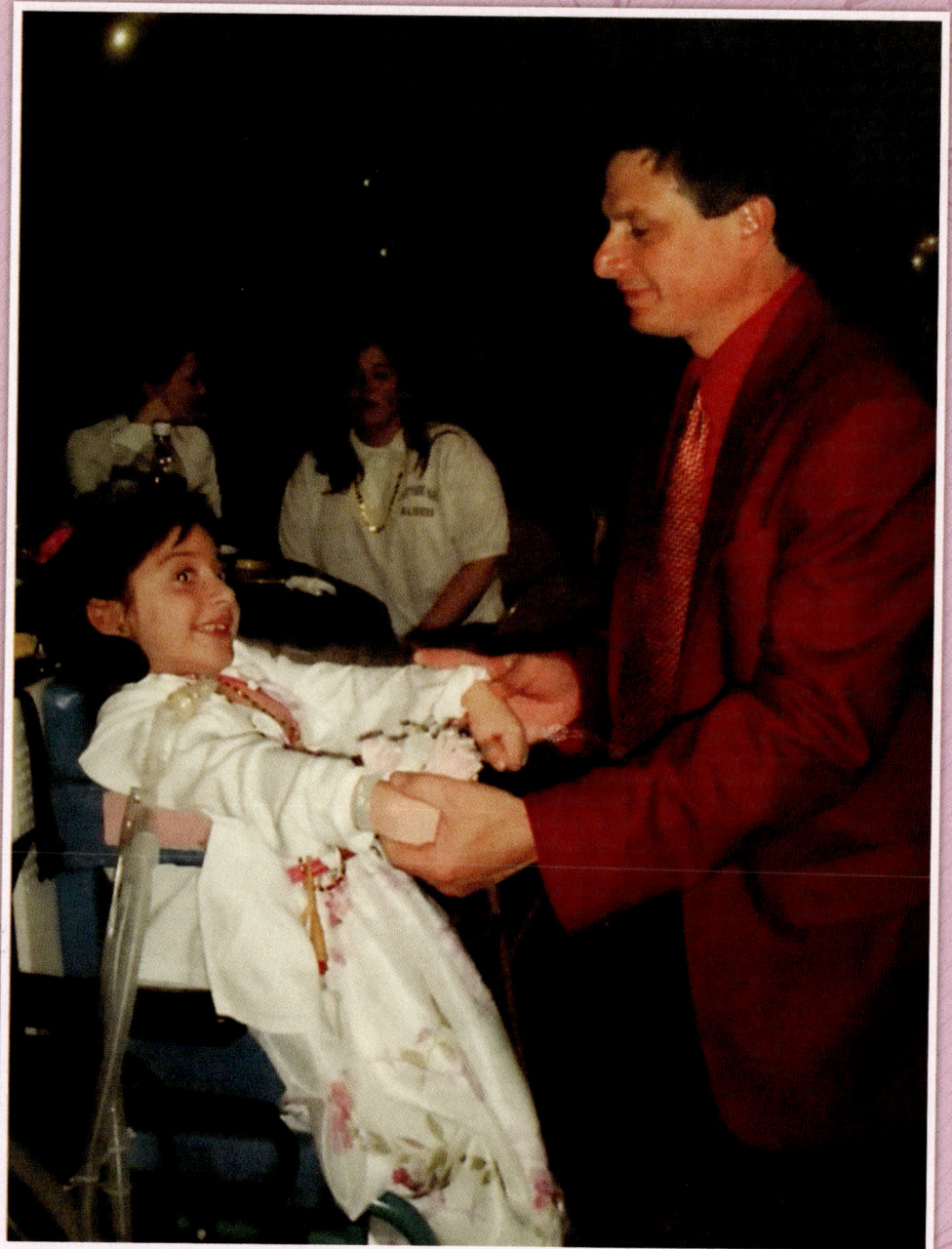
Our first daddy-daughter dance

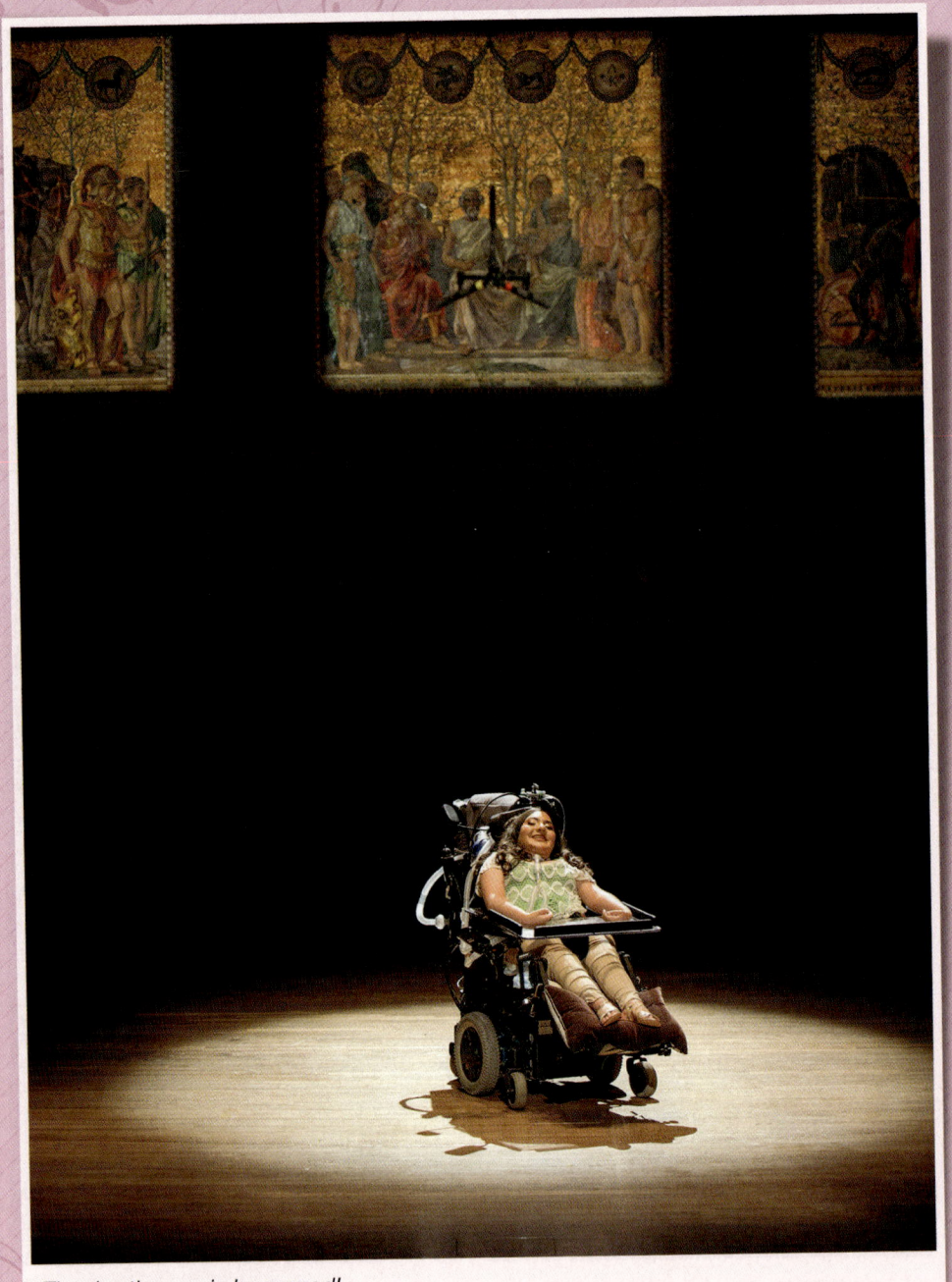
The day the magic happened!

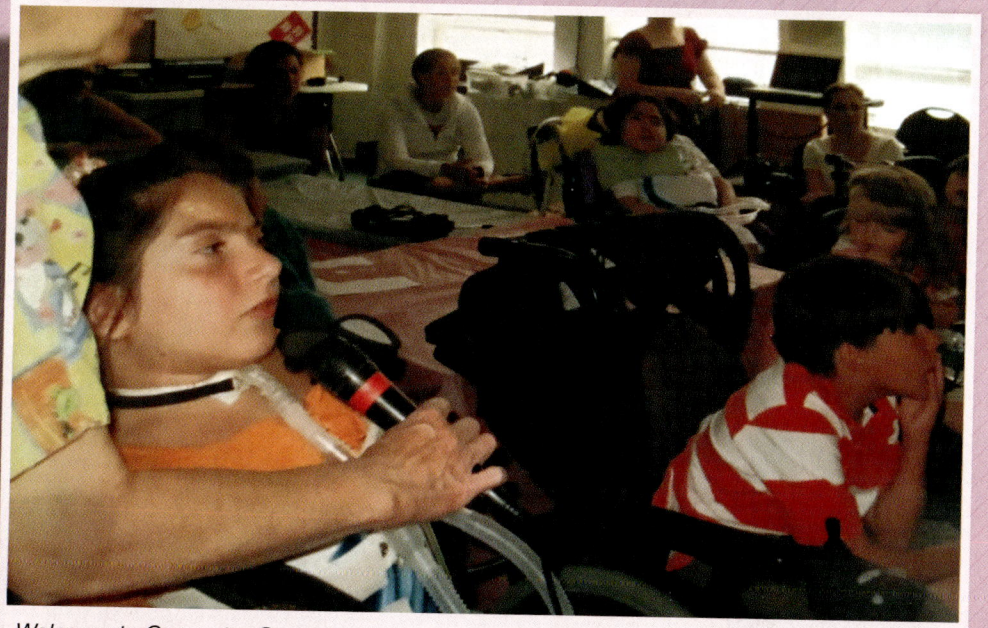
Welcome to Computer Camp Idol lol

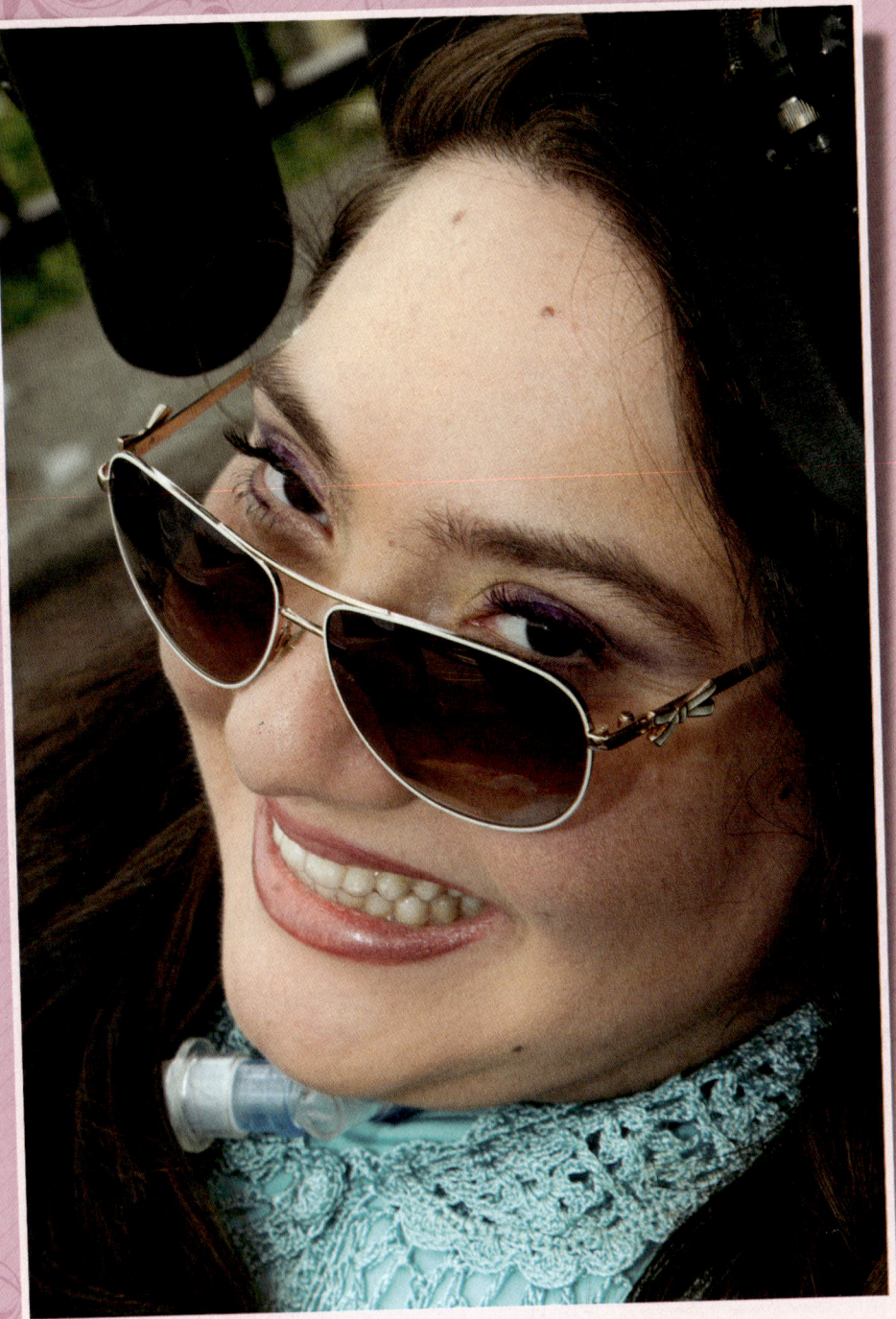
Rockin' my new shades!

Chapter 24
Inspiration

Driven by my love of music and interest in musical theater, I love to and I am determined to get out and see people perform as much as possible. I try to inspire as many people as possible because I know by helping one I am helping a million. I also get inspired, as well. I get a lot of inspiration through faith, myself, and performing. My faith inspires me to keep going and pushing and pursuing my dreams. Then, doing what I love to do inspires others and myself. Finally, watching people do what I love to do inspires me, since I can see myself one day being on that stage. In the meantime, until that dream is accomplished, I love YouTube and watching the videos being posted, and I do it all the time. But every now and then, I crave the experience of seeing a performance live, in person. This isn't always easy; I need to travel with a few people: a driver, a nurse, and a companion, at a minimum.

I need to have some very careful scouting done before I go anywhere I'm not familiar with. You'd be surprised at how many places say they are fully accessible but turn out to have a couple of steps in front of the entrance or bathroom doors that are too narrow for my chair. I am sensitive to even the slightest bumps, so I need people to watch where I am going.

The best scout and travel companion for my trips into New York City is my father. He is an expert on New York City. If I am not sure about a place, he will look into it. He spots every possible problem. When I am with him, I know I'm safe.

Even if a concert or performance location is totally accessible, it may not be ideal for me. The other audience members may crowd me, bump me, and stand between me and the stage so I can't see. I am able to elevate my chair for a better view, but the best way for me to see a show is to get special access so I can be in a spot that's not crowded. Of course, that's everyone's dream. Who wouldn't want to be able to see a show from backstage where the stars walk right next to you?

I have been to so many shows, and I have so many favorites. I have to say my favorite concerts were Maroon 5, Demi Lovato, and Justin Timberlake. All three of these artists inspire me. I remember being with one of my best friends named Ashley at Justin Timberlake's concert, and we were dancing and I was crying with excitement. Another show that was extremely memorable was Demi Lovato's. It was amazing. My neighbor Antonia went with me, and we had so much fun. Last but not least, Maroon 5. I didn't go with any of my friends; it was just my mom, my brother, my nurse, of course, and I. I started crying with excitement again. When I'm really excited, whether I'm at a party or concert, I can stay up really late, but my body will start acting up because it's tired.

Hugh Miller

"Antonia calls me 'Miller.' Not sure she knows my first name. She is the only person on the planet I let get away with this. Getting to know Antonia has been a joy for me. She is a kindred spirit. I was introduced to her and Fazi many years ago by Wade Martin, who has been a godsend to Antonia and her family. To know her is to love her. Not only is she a cool cat, she is smart as a whip, and a real ball buster.

Antonia's true love and her calling is the arts. She and I have that in common. We both love movies, books, theater, and music. And she is a wiz when it comes to pop culture. I enjoy sending Antonia to shows and concerts. From time to time she gets backstage to meet the talent. When I joined her for a concert by One Direction, the arena was filled with thousands of screaming teenage girls. While Antonia didn't scream, she was equally excited and may have enjoyed the show more than anyone.

I hear that Antonia calls me her 'agent/manager.' I like that and hope that I can live up to the task. For sure, she is talented and driven, and I have no doubt that she will fulfill her dream of being the first stage actress with a ventilator. This autobiography is a testament to her talents and abilities, and I am sure that it will make a lasting impression on all who read it.

Rock on, Antonia. I know that you will inspire so many others to overcome obstacles and achieve their goals."

Chapter 25
Performing

I'm not satisfied just seeing others perform; I want to perform, too. Sure, it's a little harder for me to perform, but I think it's hard for all performers. I love all kinds of music, and I think if I hadn't been injured, I would probably play an instrument. Singing is the only way I can make music. My voice is the only thing I can control. And I'm not in ideal condition for singing, but I do it anyway: my vocal chords can be under strain because I can't use my diaphragm, and for the most part, I'm always sitting down. *Unless I'm in the stander where singing is the easiest.*

When I first started singing, my doctors loved it. They were so proud and shocked that I had this ability, and their encouragement helped me. I hoped they liked the singing itself, but I'm pretty sure they liked how singing would get me to exercise my lungs.

If you Google me, you can find videos of me singing. I post videos on YouTube as often as I can. I do a lot of cover songs, and I hope this is good exposure and that eventually something amazing will come out of it. In the past, I could record and post a video by myself, singing a song with my sip and puff in my mouth. But YouTube has taken down its webcam feature, so now I need someone to help me.

I have had a few opportunities to sing and perform in front of live audiences, such as in the musical theater productions in high school as well as singing and speaking for certain foundations. I'm trying my best to find a way to break into show business. I think there must be some creative people out there who will help develop creative ways to incorporate me, and people like me, into their productions. I feel like society today has come a long way, but I don't think we've made it to the point to accept disabilities in show business. I hope that whether it's a year from now or five years from now, something evolves to include everyone. So far, I've had no luck. The people I have met up to now all seemed interested, or at least they looked interested, when I performed in front of them, but not ready to hire me for a job. *I haven't given up. I'm trying not to give up. I won't give up.* One of my favorite quotes is "what's the point of living if you don't take chances" from *Grease*.

Chapter 26
Technology

I use a lot of technology, obviously. Some because I have to, and some because I want to. Overall, the outcome is great, but it can be overwhelming. I love all the ways that it helps me overcome my limitations. I'd be miserable without it.

VENT

As you have read, I am on a ventilator in order to breathe. The vent has a few different parts, most of which are most often mounted on a stand near me. The first part you're likely to notice is my necklace, which is a big, clear, flexible tube attached to my neck. That tube goes back to a clear canister that is partly filled with water. The water is there to humidify the air that goes into my windpipe (trachea). If the air is not sufficiently moist, my "trach" will become dry and thick, instead of clear, and can cause a mucus plug that will block my airway and cause me to need extensive suctioning.

The vent makes a gentle whooshing sound as it breathes in and out for me. After being like this for basically my whole life, I am accustomed to the noise, except when I try to record something.

For most people, a temporary power gap or failure is a minor inconvenience; for me, it could be deadly. I can't survive without my vent. Our house has a backup generator that will keep the vent operating in case of a power failure. And if I didn't have a couple of battery options, I couldn't ever move past the reach of a power cord. If I am just going from room to room in the house or out to the front porch for a minute, we use a small, limited-life battery. If I am going on a longer expedition in the power wheelchair, I'll use a more serious battery pack that offers hours of power. These days, a lot of people look for electric outlets for their phone chargers wherever they go . . . but if I were to end up looking for outlets, it would be a lot more urgent.

In addition to the humidified air that I get from my vent, I sometimes need a little extra oxygen that I get from a special pressurized green oxygen tank. Getting a little extra oxygen can help soften or even avoid spasming. When I feel my body getting tight and getting signals that I might start spasming soon, I'll ask a nurse to hook an oxygen line up to either my vent or my ambu and that's how I roll. A little extra oxygen can also help make sure I have enough oxygen when I am in a deep sleep.

WHEELCHAIRS

Another piece of technology that's essential to me is my wheelchair. Some people in wheelchairs might talk about them the way car nuts talk about their cars. So let me give you some details about my personal, customized chairs; I have more than one chair.

Around the house, I spend most of my time in my manual (motorless) chair that people can move me around in. This chair doesn't have a battery and a motor, but it's still heavy. As I have grown, I have outgrown a few chairs. Because I spend so much time in a chair, it needs to be customized to my body so I'm comfortable. The chair also needs to be adjustable so that various parts of my body can be elevated or lowered, as needed. Of course, the chair has brakes that can lock the wheels to keep the chair from rolling. When I'm in this chair, I almost always have my table/tray in front of me, which fits right onto my chair so I can rest my hands on it more comfortably. I also keep other stuff on it often. The chair is set up so that my vent can be attached to it when I move from room to room. It also has some storage space for a few essentials, such as the oxygen if needed and my stuffed animals to help brace my position.

When I am out and about, I am most often in my power wheelchair that I can drive myself. This chair is even more customized, elaborate, and heavy. The chair's motor is electric, powered by a rechargeable battery that looks like a car battery. The controller for the chair, which looks like a remote control or a cell phone, is mounted above the end of the right hand armrest, up high enough so that I can easily see it. I give commands to the controller by inhaling or blowing into a thin straw that is positioned close enough to my mouth so that I can grab it or release it by moving my head. When I am not driving myself, someone else can control it. This chair has many features, such as elevate, recline, and tilt. When I'm not using it, the power chair stays in the garage, at the top of a ramp just outside a door from the kitchen.

ELEVATOR

There's a small elevator in the house so that I can easily be moved between the first, second, and third floors. Most of the time when I am awake I am on the first floor where it's more likely that someone will be near in case I need help.

VAN

We have a customized van with a lift that allows my power wheelchair, with me in it, to be loaded into the back of the van. Once in the van, my chair and vent can be securely locked in place. I haven't yet figured out how to control the sound system in the van, but that's OK because I usually have my own music on earphones. As long as the driver of the van avoids serious bumps and potholes, I am reasonably comfortable.

COMPUTER

To me, my computer, iPad, and cell phone technology is just as important as my vent and my chair. I have a brain that just won't quit, and I might go crazy if I didn't have ways to gain information, to learn, and to communicate. Lucky for me, I found a great technology specialist to work with. Andrew Purwin, my technology specialist, has helped me get up and running on my devices. He taught me things such as how to use a mouth stick to control my iPad and iPhone. At the same time, I have taught him about what works for me and what doesn't and what I'm interested in. I'm a fast learner, so we've also had time to hang together and be friends. In fact, he was the only one, other than my mom, who, when my depression can be really bad, I could talk about it and he would understand.

Let me tell you a little about my computer set-up. The most important part of my computer set-up is my "scan" device that lets me use the same air tube technology I use to drive my power chair to navigate and operate my computer.

The scan device places a screen within the screen. The scan screen shows me an array of things I can choose by blowing or inhaling on the tube. Often, I have to go through a sequence of steps to accomplish something that someone using a keyboard and a mouse could do much faster. Unfortunately, the makers of my scan device don't update their technology as quickly as I would like, and, as a result, my scan isn't always compatible with some of the other software installed on my computer. Even though it's not a perfect technology and it can be tiring to use, my scan enables me to operate my computer by myself. This is HUGE.

Andrew Purwin, technology consultant

"I remember the first day that we met; Antonia was just finishing up eighth grade. We were in the therapy room (if you ask Tone . . . this is referred to as HER room) at Weehawken High School. I remember walking into the room, and without warning or introductions, she started firing off questions . . . I thought to myself . . . oh, crap, this is an interview! I should have prepared better for this. I recall the first question that immediately came out of her mouth as soon as I walked through the door; she asked me, 'So . . . I hear you're a geek, huh?' I remember immediately rebutting with 'depends on what your definition of geek is.' 'If you have to ask the definition, then YOU ARE A GEEK.' I think she knew I was a geek immediately after we started talking about her iPhone . . . I guess I was speaking what she commonly refers to as 'geek talk' again.

It's funny, Antonia said to me once . . . 'I think the reason we get along so well is because you treat me like a normal girl and not a patient' . . . All I had to say to that was 'I'm not Barney Stinson from that Doogie Howser, M.D., show, and besides, you definitely are not a patient AT ALL.'

I think she is the only person at that time who would ever laugh at my corny jokes. At the time I thought she was being sympathetic; now that I've gotten to know her so well, I know she was making fun of me in her head while smirking at me behind my back.

Antonia is fearless and optimistic. When it comes to technology, she tries things on her own and works at it until she's satisfied. The only time she doesn't just go forward and waits for my help is software installation. It's really nice to work with someone who will try all these new things.

Antonia wants to be able to do things by herself. In the distant past, she had someone who would type everything for her. But she wanted to be able to do it herself. She doesn't easily accept limitations. So we have been through various softwares increasing her ability to type and to communicate with others. This is unusual. You don't generally see people in her position who have the need and drive to have that much control and independence. At this point, Antonia can control pretty much everything in the house from her iPad. With her, configuring things is always work in process.

In terms of Antonia's school experience, technology had the potential not just to enable Antonia, but also to set up better social dynamics. Antonia needs to use technology in her everyday life; when her classmates are also using that technology, it makes them more like each other. One of the things we did for her school was to provide an iPad cart that teachers could check out. It had all the apps needed to make it possible for the teacher or a student, including Antonia, to draw a problem, project it for the class to see, save the image, and share it with others. Teachers sometimes have a somewhat slower adoption rate than younger people, so Antonia didn't get the full benefit I wanted her to receive while she was in school.

Antonia always has a lot going on; this is the way she likes it, but she can handle anything you put in front of her. She juggles things with ease, in a style that you'll not see from any other human being, much less a quadriplegic. I would love to have half of her abilities. She's the most willing person to jump into a new situation. She always wants to be doing something and has a passion for learning. If I had half of her desire to better herself, I'd be CEO of a major corporation.

Technology is our common ground, but my friendship with Antonia involves a lot more than technology. We have a close relationship . . . we just connect. She's easy to relate to, and her personality is so outgoing. When I visit her, our conversation ranges from what needs fixing in the house to what's going on in our lives; obviously, she's the more intelligent one in the conversation, but I try to keep up.

I have to add mention about Fazila, Antonia's mother. I have never seen a more loving and dedicated mother in my entire life. From the moment I met her, her entire life seems to rotate around the happiness of her children. She has more patience then any person I have ever met, and the unconditional love she has for both of her children is heartwarming. But her biggest character trait is her strength: her ability to put on a smile after both she and Antonia had been up all night because of her spasms; her ability to fold the laundry and make dinner after lifting Antonia from her stander and putting her into her wheelchair. That is the definition of character in its purest form. The ability to overcome all obstacles you put in front of her and just be grateful that whatever religious beliefs you had that somehow Antonia was saved; Fazila has never taken that for granted.

Lastly, I have to thank Wade Martin. I can see Antonia reading this and already rolling her eyes at me, but Wade is the reason I was able to meet Antonia. Wade showed me what true inspiration really is when he introduced us. I feel like this may be a repetitive statement in the story of Antonia, but if you knew her, then you would understand why everyone says knowing her is a gift because she inspires people to be better and do better (or she'll kick your butt if you don't)."

Chapter 27
Neighbors

We got lucky when we moved to the town we currently live in because the people who live next door to us are great neighbors and friends. My brother and I like to go over there and visit, and our neighbors are comfortable in our home. One of them is named Antonia and is my age. I'm just two months older than she is. So we like to joke around about being long lost, psychological twins. I'm the good twin who plays by the rules . . . most of the time. She's the evil twin who is more rebellious and socially exposed than I am. The youngest child in that family, Gianna, is my brother's age and grade. So they're like our mirror family. They understand, to an extent, what it's like growing up with a disability because the second oldest child in their family, Giselle, has Down syndrome. They help us a lot. They drive my brother to and from school. Antonia helps out when I don't have a nurse, which is relaxing because we can just hang out and be ourselves.

It's nice to have friends whom you have met by chance, not just through a special program, like some of the kids I grew up with. Not all of them were bad. Some showed respect and kindness, like Ashley and Antonia, and some of my friends from Cliffside Park, like Arwa and Stephanie. We bring complementary talents to the friendship. Those whom I spend time with keep me up-to-date about what's going on.

Chapter 28
Friends

I was chatting with my friends yesterday. Here's my depression telling me, "Oh, you're gone; they don't care about you anymore. You skipped ahead to the grade that you should have been in, and they stopped caring about you. Oh, they pretended to like you just out of pity."

But then there's the light side that says they just don't know how to act around me. Because I always have a nurse around me, so we can't always be who we want to be, but some of them just don't care, we just talk. "What have you been up to? How is college?" "I'm not in college. I'm doing what I love to do and working my way into the arts business. I've been going to auditions, meetings, here, there, and I recorded my own album. I just need to find somebody to produce it and find out if I'm on the right track." It makes me really happy and it eases the depression when I hear my friends say things like: "Girl, I'm so happy that you are following your dreams." "Don't worry, I will show up. I didn't forget about you, as long as you didn't forget about me."

One of my friends and I think exactly alike. He is funny and straight to the point, like I am. When my depression was at its worst, I would see him and a few other kids that would lighten my day. Although he and I would speak alike and joke around and say we could be miserable together. There are so many people that I met, but certain ones are real. Like I said before, whoever is true, they will come back to you.

Ashley Acevedo

"I've known Antonia since I was in fifth grade. We were in the same grade from fifth through tenth. Then Antonia skipped her junior year and went from tenth grade into twelfth. We stayed good friends even though we were in different grades. Now, we're still good friends even though she has graduated and I'm still in high school.

We have a lot in common. To start with, we both love music and acting. I see her about once a month. I go to her house, and we hang out. We talk girl stuff. We watch movies. We talk about the people we both know at school. Just like all people our age do.

Antonia is a great listener with a strong memory. If I tell her about something going on in my life, she's likely to remind me of previous experiences and reactions that I had. She gives me good advice. It's helpful. She tells me about how things are going for her and what she's thinking about. She can be emotional because of the position that she has been put in. It's not easy. Antonia will always crack a joke. She'll be sarcastic. That's part of her personality. It's part of why she's so much fun to be with."

Chapter 29
Love

Next stop . . . LOVE! Yes, I too have been in love. I think, unfortunately, most people are afraid to love someone with a disability. From puppy love in elementary school, then learning about real love in high school, and finally admitting that you are in love with someone you may or may not be able to be with are feelings everyone goes through. Just because a person has a disability doesn't mean they can't or don't feel all those things, too.

I had my first love, but unfortunately, it did not work out. I felt for him, but he did not feel for me. Like most girls, it felt like a knife was stabbing into my heart. It left this unbearable ache and this scar on my heart and mind. Unlike most girls, they have not been through most of the things that I have been through, so for them, letting go of a loved one seems impossible. I am not saying that for me it is any easier, but I learned not to get attached so fast and to try to let things go. The saying "If you love someone, set them free" is true — but unfortunately, it is so damned hard! The worst part was that I knew this person so well, and what my head was telling me is not something he would think, but I felt like he could not love me because of my injury. It may hurt like hell, but eventually it gets better. Now, Alhamdulillah, I don't have as much heartache anymore. He and I are still really good friends, and I want what's best for him. I am, for the most part, selfless and realistic. I want whoever is around me to do whatever it takes to make them happy. I know he is happy, and that makes me happy. I am realistic because I have my faith and I know that if someone is supposed to be with me, it will happen. Like the song goes, "Que Sera Sera, Whatever Will Be, Will Be." I'm not in a rush.

Chapter 30
Mental Illness

I am at a point in my life where I cannot "accept" my injury, but I can manage with it. I will never be completely okay with living like this. That is where the anxiety and depression come in. I constantly worry about my life, whether it's past, present, or future. I have these uncontrollable and constant feelings of guilt, anger, and fear. The older I get and the more I understand my life, the PTSD comes in and the memories and flashbacks of constantly being told that everything is my fault, my parents fighting, when my father's illness first started coming out, feels like it is always happening. However, I know it is all in my head. I try so hard to control these uncontrollable thoughts and feelings. I can get to the point where I feel so alone, hopeless, scared, and angry. Then on my good days, which are most days thanks to some of my medication, I feel like I can manage my life and everything happens for a reason.

I've mentioned mental illness and depression, in particular. This is a hard topic that needs to be spoken about. People are often a lot more understanding about physical injury than they are about mental illness. This is a problem. Because when people are reluctant to talk about mental illness, the individuals who are suffering think that they are all alone. They are too embarrassed and afraid to talk, thinking no one will understand them and this can make the illness get worse. That's part of why I am so open about what goes on both physically and mentally.

Just as I don't know exactly what mental illness my father suffers from, I don't know exactly what the technical terms for my mental illnesses are. I've mentioned PTSD. I've mentioned a tendency to feel guilt for things that I may not be responsible for. I've shown that I can sometimes feel paranoid and think that people are out to get me. I've said that while I can't do much with my body, my brain is hyperactive. I can become tremendously depressed.

I'm not sure which of these feelings are appropriate, given my situation. One thing that brings my anxiety and depression out is when I have nobody around me to help me with my needs, from simple things like giving me water or putting the straw that I use to type back in my mouth.

I need to have people to help me, and I need those people to be positive. This was part of the problem in school: a lot of the people around me weren't positive. I can't take it when people are tired or cranky or distressed. If you're in a bad mood, either talk it out with me or fake a smile. I can't deal with both my pain and the pains of others. I can't have someone who's angry around me because then I don't know what to do with myself. I need positive energy so I don't feel guilty, so I don't focus on the negative. My mind needs to constantly be busy. If I'm stressed out, my mind goes all over the place, more than it already is.

I don't know if all of these issues are due to the injury or due to what my father could possibly have. I also don't know how to factor in the effects of my injury and of all the medications I need to take. Medications definitely affect my brain and my mood. And let's call the medications what they are: my drugs. It's a rougher sounding word but appropriate. To make things even harder, the "sweet spot" for drugs is a moving target. I can find what I think is the right combination and dosage, but after a while, my body and brain won't be as responsive to them.

My life right now is finally starting to go in the direction that I want it to. I am still adjusting to going out in public and meeting casting directors, managers, and agents. The anxiety comes out when I am at these meetings because part of me still feels like I do not fit in a public setting. I know this is not true. Even though I get very anxious when I'm at an audition, I always try my hardest to not let it stop me.

Chapter 31
Sadness

I still have sadness, a sadness that is like an animal trying to break out of a cage. If I don't get my mind under control, it can turn into an unforeseen form of depression . . . one that controls who I am and how I see the world. It forces me to analyze every moment of every minute of every day. This makes me want to scream and cry out at the same time. It turns me dark, into a mere glimmer of the person I expect myself to be. I feel like no one sees me as who I am. This tortuous pain evolves into an emptiness. I feel as though no matter what is said and done, there is nothing that can fill the void that is creating this loneliness and sadness.

The first few years after the accident were not easy; in fact, it was a really dark and confusing time for all of us. Between the ages of three and seven, very few people understood me. I remember feeling so sad and alone during those years.

The awareness of how different I had become weighed heavily on my family. I started to realize how vulnerable and unable to protect myself I was. I grew fearful of the pain that people could cause by just bumping into me. I began to think, at moments, that some people were even bumping into me because they didn't care. I started to dread social contact and to prefer isolation.

I began to feel that I was somehow responsible for many of the bad things that were happening to my family. Today I understand intellectually that it's silly and perhaps egotistical for a young child to feel responsibility and guilt for things beyond her control. But once these feelings appeared, they sent out deep roots. I can't seem to totally eliminate them. Every now and then, they reappear and try to grow. Some of it I can control and some of it I can't. The guilt that I can't control hurts me, and, as you have read, it causes my depression. However, as you have read, there are two things that have the power to ease some of the sadness: Islam and music.

Chapter 32
PTSD

When I tell people that I suffer from PTSD, they often look at me strangely. PTSD (Post-Traumatic Stress Disorder) is a term that is most often used for soldiers, hostages, and residents of devastated areas who have ongoing mental and emotional difficulties in the aftermath of battles that they have been in. In many cases, thanks to adrenaline, they performed well during the emergencies but found themselves shaken and changed as they continued to process what they did and endured. The people who don't look at me strangely often make the assumption that the trauma that caused my PTSD was the car collision that caused my injury.

Actually, I think the greater trauma, and the cause of my PTSD, is what I experienced throughout my life and in school. As you have read earlier, my chiropractor Alek said something that is very hard for me to admit to. I bury a lot of feelings and emotions very deep down inside. You have to understand how different and difficult my life can be. I can feel completely exposed. There is no way to keep anything private. I get extremely fearful. I feel defenseless. In school, I desperately wanted to participate but wasn't given the chance. Instead, I was pushed until I spasmed and cried and interrupted everything. *That wasn't the kind of attention I wanted.* I had no control over anything. I felt like I was being tortured and publicly ridiculed day after day after day.

Now, as a young adult, I am still thinking of these bad memories. I feel like a broken record because they can go on and on in my head. They make me cautious and suspicious. They can make me reluctant to try new groups and environments. They fuel my feelings of paranoia. Overall, that's how my mind can get. On my good days, I feel mostly mentally stable; however, feelings of anger and agitation rarely leave me.

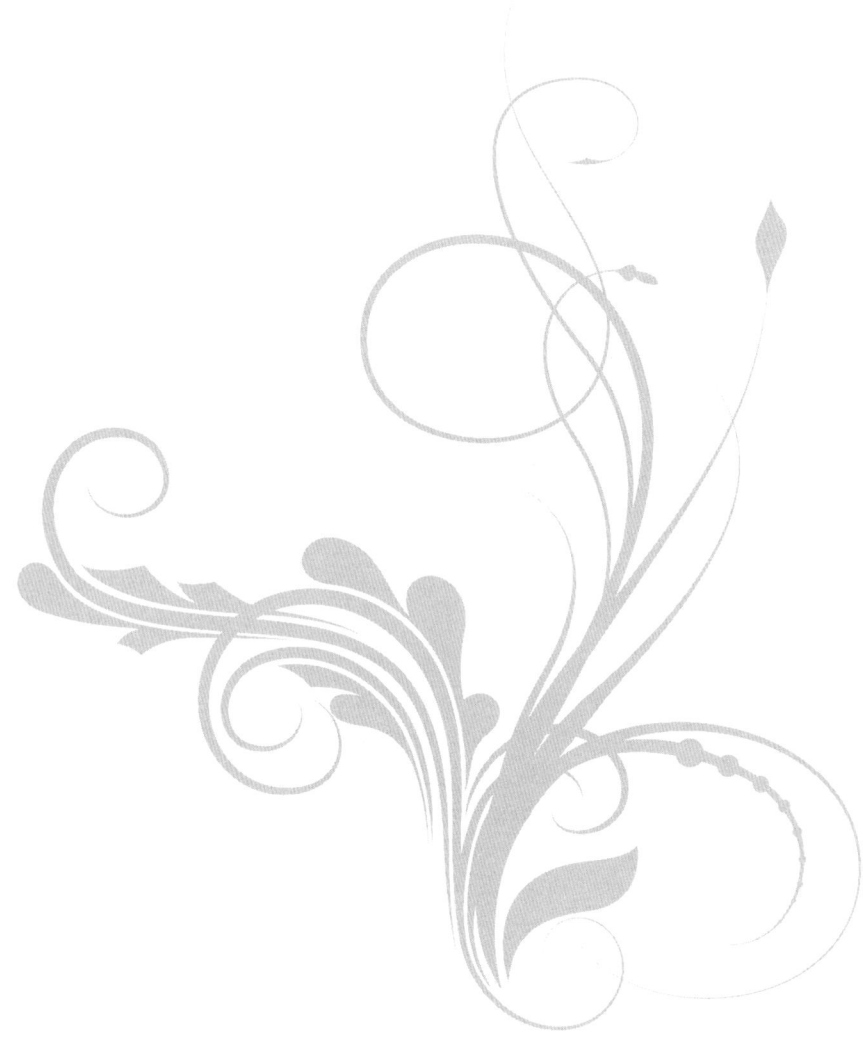

Chapter 33
High School

The more I stayed in high school, the more I lost myself. There's a lack of mutual respect and effort on the part of some people in that school. I tried to last six years, but I couldn't take it anymore. Not just the school part, but also my body couldn't handle it anymore. I started feeling like I was pushing myself too hard.

During the school years, I started off being polite and cautious in how I spoke to people and always tried to make everyone happy, first by saying, "Excuse me, excuse me, excuse me," as I made my way through the hallways and being extremely passive about everything that went on. Eventually, the frustrations of everyday life and constant pain would prompt me to shout, "Yo! Idiot, MOVE" or "Hey! Watch where you're going." *(My motto is "Treat everybody with respect; give them three chances: first time, nice; second time, firm; third time, show them I mean business.")*

Another problem: people would exclude me. In high school, teachers and students were likely to start into a lesson or project without involving me. They just didn't make the extra effort that was needed so I could contribute. But this just wasn't fair. It can be near impossible for me to catch up when I haven't been involved from the beginning. I can be a slow learner if you don't know how to teach or work with me the right way.

I would try to participate in a social environment as much as possible; but, depending on who was in it, I might get ignored. Sometimes I would come up to a group engaged in a conversation and ask them what they were talking about, only to be completely ignored and blocked out. Sometimes, depending on the situation, I would think, "Hello! Are you blind? I'm right here." Or, if I were flustered enough, I would actually say it.

Being excluded bothered me all the more because we had made it possible through my personal funding to equip the school and the teachers with all sorts of technology and tools to make it easier to involve me and make the school more up-to-date for the students. We put in Wi-Fi, installed Smart Boards and provided iPads. But often the teachers didn't seem interested in using the technology *(except they seemed to enjoy using the iPads for personal business and wanted to hang on to them)*.

Throughout my education, I generally had my own personal teacher or aide with me, and I would have thought that they would have helped me stand up for myself when necessary. Unfortunately, 90 percent of the time, it worked the other way. When I wanted to speak up, they shushed me. One of the things they said when they wanted to keep me quiet was "I'm a professional. This is my job. I know what's best for you because I have special degrees, qualifications, and experience." "I know what's best for you" is a sentence I HATE hearing from anyone except my mother, and some of my nurses. The only person who truly knows me is Allah, my mother, and I.

These adults knew next to nothing about my body or my injury. They may have earned some sort of certificate from the state, but they certainly hadn't learned much about asking questions, listening, or empathy. They, and many people in this world, were and are under the illusion that all special needs students were essentially the same. In fact, each of us is unique. Until a person comes to understand that, he or she will be unable to help individualize education programs and make them appropriate for someone who has unique needs. As much as you have read about my educational experience, I have to admit that it could have been much better, but it could have been a hell of a lot worse.

Rob Ferullo

"You can't have a bad day around Antonia. She's positive, inspiring, and basically unbreakable.

I worked with Antonia for six years, helping design her school programs. It was always complicated but was an amazing opportunity. Antonia's team was ready to provide the resources that the school needed to be able to address Antonia's needs.

When designing the program, all variables had to be considered: the size and weight of her chair; noise from the vent; the two extra adults in every room. (Antonia had a private teacher as well as an ER-level nurse specialized in trauma.) We had to go through the process of selecting the appropriate teacher. In addition, we had to design an emergency plan to remove Antonia from the building in the event of a catastrophic building failure, such as a fire, that resulted in no electricity or elevator. Every room Antonia used needed to have air conditioning, so we tried to double up room usage when possible.

The teachers would always have to have Antonia near the exits for safety purposes. She would often have to leave her classroom early to get to the next class on time because of the speed of the chair. Also, Antonia had her own private room with a bathroom because of the needs she had. When Antonia became exhausted, she would go to her room to rest.

Antonia wanted to be involved in everything possible. She was in the play and joined the mock trial. She was exempt from gym, but that made sense and seemed more than fair, given how much she had to put into just navigating through her day.

While we made some accommodations for Antonia, she and her team always asked that she be treated like everyone else as much as possible. They invested in making this possible, providing air conditioning and technology such as Smart Boards. Since iPads were the best way to optimize Antonia's education, her team provided them for every teacher every year. I would then organize iPad training for those teachers.

Synergy is an overused word, but in this case, it's the right word. We really had a lot of synergy across our whole team. Everybody was on the same page, and that synergy started with her. I enjoyed working with Antonia and her family. They guided us through it all and provided tremendous feedback. The shared goals and inspiration continued through her other team members, including Wade Martin and Andrew Purwin. Her care managers and her nurses all deserve credit. Her private teacher, Mr. Coffaro, played a critical role in school and as a liaison with her team at home.

The synergy extended to a broad team within the school. Everybody was inspired and stepped up to the challenge. I think it would be hard not to want the best for

Antonia. There was never a moment when I said to myself, 'Let's not bother with this next step or this extra effort.' After all, I knew it took her an hour and a half working with multiple adults just to get ready for school each morning . . . so how could I let myself, or any member of her team, underdeliver.

While there are many people who deserve credit, no one deserves more credit than Antonia herself. She has modeled herself on her mother, who is an amazingly strong woman. In the face of all of the challenges that Antonia faces, she remains determined and positive. How could anyone not respond to that?"

Chapter 34
Two Proms!

Because I skipped eleventh grade, I ended up feeling like I was a member of two different classes: the high school graduating classes of 2015 and 2016. I was always with the class of 2016, but then I graduated with the class of 2015. Either way, both classes of kids are my family. I've met some really good kids whom I love, and that's why the class of 2016's prom was the more emotional one.

When I completed my senior year in 2015, I graduated and went to the prom. The theme was Mardi Gras. We all dressed up and had a great time. I think I stayed out until almost midnight — it was awesome that my body allowed me to stay out that late. Because I had just joined the class of 2015 in their senior year, my mind made me think that they didn't care about me at all; but prom night made me realize I was wrong.

When the members of the class of 2016 — who had been my classmates through tenth grade — started thinking about their prom, a few of them started asking me if I would be there. I told them that my heart wanted to be there, but I wasn't sure if I was allowed to because I was no longer a student at the school and didn't think I would be allowed to go to prom. Finally, our wish came true. Thanks to some of the staff, the school said yes. Sometime later, they found me a date to go to prom with. Of course, getting ready for a prom is never simple. My mom and I went shopping for another dress. A lot of text messages went back and forth as to where we would meet. The girls and I were getting even more excited than we already were.

Now the hard part: getting dressed and ready. Getting dressed is not easy for me. My spasms always interfere, so my mom and I had to relax my body as much as we could, and, Alhamdulillah, we managed to get the dress on. Then later, the fun stuff — the hair, makeup, and accessories — were all done by my nurse.

The music at the prom was mostly Latin music, but I don't care as long as I'm driving my chair with the people I love. That's all I care about. It was fun to move my chair and dance with everybody. I felt a special joy at seeing how suddenly grown up many of my former classmates seemed. It was very weird but awesome at the same time because after a year of not being in the school, everyone looked so grown up and matured. It wasn't just the fancy clothing, although that helped. It was also great to see the people whom I had first met as awkward young kids now happily in couples. I was also thrilled that even though some of the kids were half of a couple, they still danced with me as if nothing has changed. Because, to me, I feel like nothing should or did change. It's PROM. That's supposed to mean the one and last night where everybody is together. It felt nice and heartbreaking at the same time. I hope that we will keep in touch through social media, FaceTime, etc., or, hopefully, the future will bring us together again. On the surface, I am 90 percent hard as steel, but inside I'm a blob. I love (most of) the kids I met from Cliffside Park, Bergen County Special Services, and Weehawken Classes of 2016 and 2015. I can't wait to see what the future holds for us.

Chapter 35
Finding the Right College

As it turns out, relatively few colleges are ready to accept a student in my situation. Not only do they have to believe that I can do the work, but they also have to be ready to welcome my entourage — my nurse and an aide or teacher who come along with me. To accept me, a college has to be confident that they can make their facilities accessible to me and willing to accept the challenge, something that's not always easy. They have to be ready to embrace the digital technology I require. They know that they will need to review their evacuation and safety programs. They need to be willing to address any professors or instructors who might not be prepared to do the extra work to make it possible for me to participate. You get the idea. Accepting me as a student is a big commitment. Although it's the kind of commitment that colleges will need to make more and more going forward.

At first, I was rejected by a few colleges. This was depressing and devastating to me because it made me feel like I was rejected because of my injury. My confidence went downhill, but in the end, everything is worth it. I ended up doing what I originally wanted to do. I took a year off and started my career and focused on my body. I am a determined person and, for the most part, do not take no for an answer, so even though it's a competitive world out there, I applied to different schools again. Just when I was starting to feel discouraged and anxious, I was flabbergasted when I got the news that I was accepted to a college. I couldn't believe that a school actually wanted me to go. It's going to take a lot of effort to make it work; however, I'm eager for this challenge. I've got a lot of hopes and ambitions, and having a college education could help me achieve them. My dad would always say, "aspetta un momento" or "just wait a minute" in Italian. I am not in a rush. I know it is going to be hard, and I know my future is going to be even harder. I am going to take one step at a time.

Chapter 36
Ongoing Challenges

When you are severely injured as a young child, doctors need to fix your body periodically to accommodate growth, unlike adults who have already reached full growth. In the accident, my neck was broken, so they had to fuse the bones together. First they put in a wire to fuse the bones. As I grew, the wire wasn't growing with me. I felt like this wire was trying to poke out of my neck, and it was putting pressure on some of the nerves. This caused more spasms that were EXTREMELY painful and long. The doctors took that out, and I wore a neck brace for several months.

Then the doctors realized that my curvature was really bad; my spine was curling into a "C" position. So, to ease some of my pain at the time, they redid the fusing of my upper spine, adding steel for support. They could have fused more of my spine, but I don't want that. *At least not yet.* I am trying alternative options.

I have grown since then, so I could have another surgery, but I am not in the mood for any surgery right now. *Ain't nobody got time for that.*

Chapter 37
Taking Control

Over the years, I have learned to take more and more control over my medical treatment. I read up on every medication I take, and I generally know not only what they do, but also how they do it. I do so much research on the Internet that my neurosurgeon told me, "If you really want to be a doctor, I'll help you."

I have respect for doctors, especially the ones that really care. But, ultimately, I know my body best. If I'm sick, or overheated or in a bad position, my body is going to act out. When you are a newly injured girl, you don't know what you need. You're confused. What you need are people who are willing to listen. If a physical therapist is bending your leg, and you say you can't breathe, you need someone who is listening or willing to listen. The people who are treating the patient need to work with the patient. They need to follow the patient's lead. And that's what my chiropractor mostly does. I say, "I have pain here, here, and here in my body." And he'll work in that area. Often this can be painful, so I will tell him to go slowly, and he listens.

For the most part, I am picky about my caregivers. For example, I can tell whether or not someone is strong enough to work with my body. If you're not strong enough, it will be too hard for you to control my spasms. Same with doctors. I don't care how many degrees you have, or where you give guest lectures. None of that matters if you don't have time to see me, talk to me, and work with me. *Hey, we are the only ones who know our bodies.* The doctors know the basics of how the body is programmed. But when you live with it, you learn more than the basics. I need help for my body, yes. Focusing on my pain is not going to do me any good. I need to multitask. I've always been good at multitasking. Whoever you are, be the authority on you.

I decided that I needed to take more control over my own medical treatment, and I saw that there was some hope for improvement; the next logical step was for me to improve my overall health.

I've become a health nut about what I consume. When I was younger, food and drink did not affect my body, so I could eat and drink whatever I wanted. As I got older, I had to start watching what I ate. I try to eat healthy foods as much and as often as I can. As I get older, my injury causes more complications such as frequent bladder spasms and incontinence. I do what I can to keep my bladder calm by avoiding caffeinated beverages.

I rely on a combination of the right foods, vitamins, and Ensure, a liquid nutritional supplement, to stay strong. I need the Ensure because my body needs extra nutritional support. Without Ensure, I'd become weak fairly quickly. I require a ton of vitamins. When I eat a lot of greens, I don't have to take all my vitamins or Ensure. So I drink lots of blended-up greens.

I also try to get enough exercise. I have a therapeutic exercise bike. I hook up electrodes to the muscles of my leg, and they give them stimulation to make my legs move. I like it when the machine shows that my body is doing the work because it shows that it is waking up. I hope to get handles for the bike so I can do the same thing for my arms. Right now, my mom and a few other people exercise my arms. I also exercise by just standing for increasing periods of time. The more I move, the better for my body because the pins and needles, which contribute to spasms, ease.

Chapter 38
Hope

Members of my family have always told me, "Allah made you like this for a reason." Most of my life I did not believe or accept this. I have come to embrace this situation. This is my destiny. I don't know precisely what it is yet, but I do know that I need to keep searching for it. I may not accomplish all I set out to do, but that is expected for everybody. There is value in me trying. It's like the song "The Impossible Dream" in the musical *Man of La Mancha*.

I want to be the first person in show business with a severe spinal cord injury and ventilator. There's a surgery in which a doctor can implant a device in the diaphragm called a pulmonary pacemaker. That's my dream. If I can't accomplish that, then I want to inspire people one way or another. I believe that everybody has a voice, including people with disabilities, so I try to speak for the voiceless.

I wouldn't mind giving guest lectures on spinal cord injuries, drunk driving, or mental illness. I can testify from my own experience about how music has the ability to reach people and open them up. Music can open more doors in you than anything else. You can listen to the lyrics. You can listen to the melody or feel it, whatever works for each person. Music can heal. Among my many dreams, one of them is to become a music therapist. Whatever I do, it has to somehow involve music.

I also like the idea of regaining the parts of my heritage that have been lost. I would like to learn the Italian language, culture, and cuisine that weren't passed on to us. I have such a strong embrace on my Guyanese culture from my mother's side. I feel that if I regain some of the Italian side, I will be closing a gap that I feel, and this will strengthen the ties to my father and his side of the family.

As I've already indicated, I dream of the same things that many typical people dream of. I'd like to get married and have children. For that matter, if Allah wills it and someday I get married and I am able to spend significant stretches of time off my vent, I dream that my husband and I might take a month off and travel Italy from top to bottom. *See how all these dreams link up with each other?*

Sure, they're just dreams. And I may have told myself a time or two that I wouldn't write a book . . . well, you're reading my book that I wrote right now. I want to show the world that there's more to everything and to keep an open mind. Dreams can come true.

Another ambition of mine is helping other people by sharing some of what I have learned on my journey so far. Sharing with you what I've learned so far, in the hopes that it might be helpful.

Chapter 39
Find Inspiration

I work hard to stay inspired. I need to stay inspired and not let the darkness control me. I find a lot of inspiration in songs. One song that moves me is "Shadow Days" by John Mayer. He sings,

*"I'm a good man, with a good heart
Had a tough time, got a rough start
But I finally learned to let it go
Now I'm right here, and I'm right now
And I'm hoping, knowing somehow
That my shadow days are over now."*

I relate to everything he is saying, except the part about being a man . . . *obviously*. This song inspires me because it's not easy for someone to admit that they have darkness in them. It makes me happy to hear someone singing about putting their darkness behind them.

Another song that gets to me is "Human" by Christina Perri. She sings,

*"I can do it
But I'm only human
And I bleed when I fall down
I'm only human
And I crash and I break down
Your words in my head, knives in my heart
You build me up and then I fall apart
'Cause I'm only human."*

She expresses how much you can get hurt by other people when you try to please them and how much words and actions can hurt. I know what she's talking about. Many people, especially around my age, are not accepting of themselves. They are dealing with many issues internally, and that is a problem that I still struggle with.

I'm inspired by Angela Rockwood, a model/actress who suffered a spinal cord injury similar to mine but not as severe in a car accident, and many of the girls from the television show *Push Girls*. *Push Girls* is a reality TV series about four women with various levels of paralysis living in Hollywood, California. The show only lasted two seasons, but it was a breakthrough, especially for me. It inspired me and gave me hope. Whatever you're facing, find things that inspire you so you have the strength to keep going.

Chapter 40
Learn to Accept Help

Learning to accept help has been one of the hardest lessons I've learned throughout my journey, and I hate admitting it. Of course, I have no choice. But it still frustrates me. I'm a take-charge person by nature. In school, I would be the head of the team on most projects, and I would get after team members who were not pulling their weight. I inherited a certain amount of impatience from each of my parents. If I hadn't been injured, I'm sure I would do almost everything by myself.

I am naturally an observer. I know that other people need help. No person can do everything by themselves. I want to help the people that I love and care about, but I am limited, so I can't do as much as I would like. The best way to help people is by paying it forward, and there are so many ways to do that. A lot of people help me. And I, in turn, look for ways to help others, mainly by inspiring people. *Hey, at least I'm trying.*

Other than paying it forward, the best thing to do is be humble and kind. I am trying to be both of those things even if it can be very hard . . . *I'm working on it.*

Chapter 41
Believe in Something Bigger than Yourself

My faith keeps me going. When my depression was at its peak, I had very little faith. But I did have a little. I deliberately enlarged that faith because I knew I shouldn't feel the way I was feeling. I had too much crap in my head, and it was blocking me from doing the things that I needed to be doing and thinking the way that I needed to think. It worked. By expanding my faith, I found a way to counterbalance the depression.

One way I increase my faith is by listening to Islamic lectures and music. If I come across something that I think people should know, I will share it (mostly on Facebook). I particularly like Nouman Ali Khan and Dr. Zakir Naik. They helped me when I was confused. Their lectures continue to help me. When you have problems, they can seem so big that you'll never be able to overcome them. By believing in something bigger than yourself, you can tap into a power even bigger than your problems. It also helps you stay open-minded and realize you are not alone.

Chapter 42
Never Give Up

If you give up, you'll never know what you could have done. I was told I would always be 100 percent dependent on my vent, but I learned that with practice that is not true. Now I am working slowly but surely to increase the time I can be off the vent. No one thought it was possible to sing while on a vent either, but obviously I am succeeding.

Here's an example. My friend Rachel from Bergen County Special Services has had limited relief when it came to her spasms for as long as I have known her. In recent years, she has had an operation and has worked amazingly hard on her own rehabilitation. She has made great strides and continues to show vast improvements on her typing and her walking. Her spirit continues to inspire me, and I am so proud of her.

I'm going to try my hardest to inspire people as well to do what I love to do. It may be hard. It may be annoying. But I'm sure as hell not going to give it up. Even if something is not possible, I am going to try to make it possible.

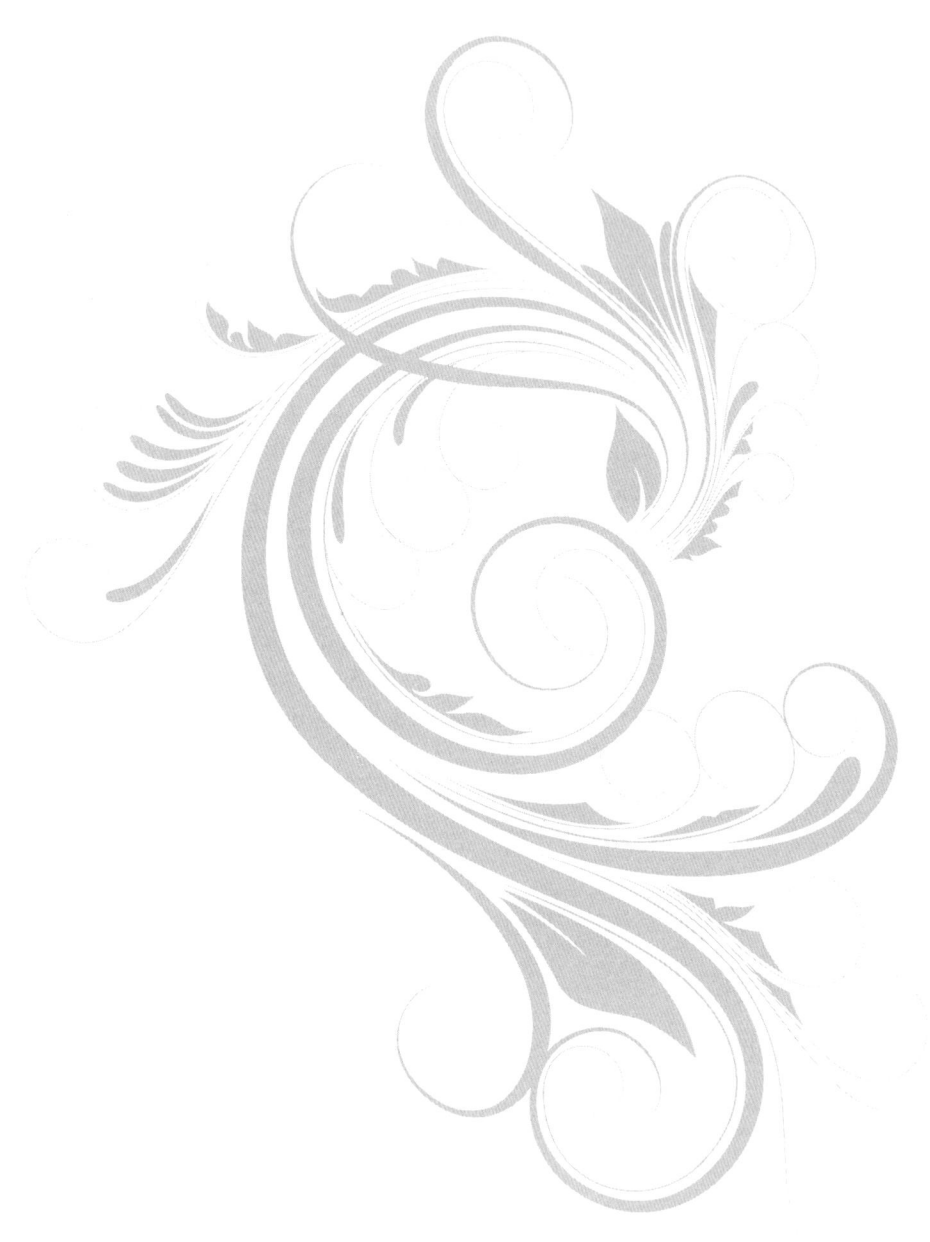

Chapter 43
Be Different

I love to see or hear about people who are not afraid to be different. I love outspoken people who stand up and speak out for what they believe in. I find it inspiring when people are true to themselves. Individuality, artistic flair, and those who always hold on to their humanity inspire me!

When I think about the people, and particularly the artists, that I like, I realize that they each are willing to be just a little different from the mainstream, and they are open about how they are different. There are so many artists who inspire me, but for the sake of this book, I will only list a few.

Lady Gaga, in addition to being a terrific performer, has been open about her rape ordeal as a teenager. She has spoken to the hearts of those in a similar situation as her and has helped countless individuals cope with their situation. Those who have the audacity to inspire are the ones who teach us to inspire others. She dedicated "Till It Happens to You" to millions of people. She does not sing just one style; she stays true to herself musically.

Harry Connick Jr. is a jack of all genres, which I respect *and hopefully will be*. He also acts, both on stage and on the big screen. He composes as well. He is another one who shows true talent and artistry.

Josh Groban is so talented he could sing in any format. Instead of focusing on best-selling pop, he performs in a wide variety of styles, including operatic singing.

You may face particular challenges, but there's no reason to let your challenges be the only thing that's different about you. Be willing to follow your own curiosity into the areas that make you special. When my depression is at its worst, I tell myself "normal is boring," and I believe that most of the time. If you think about it this way, if God wanted us to "be normal," everybody and everything would be the same.

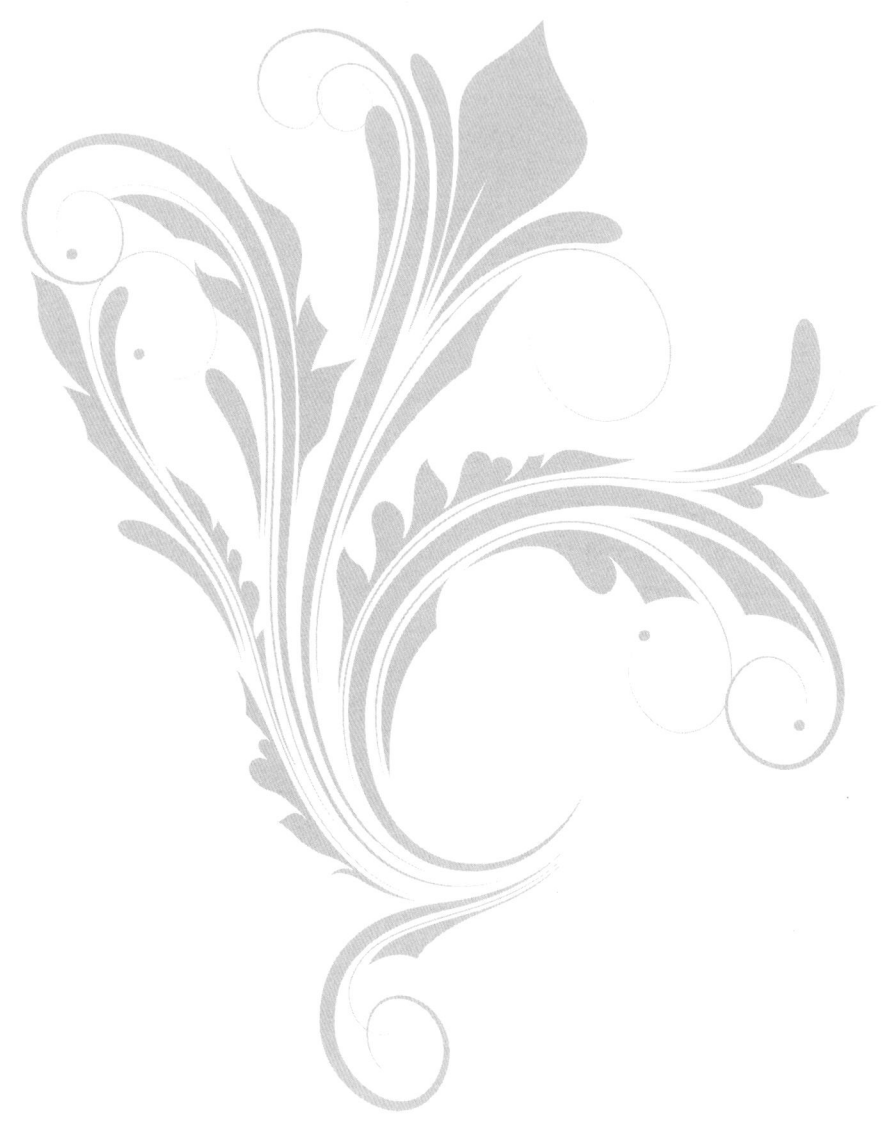

Chapter 44
Speak Up

People can't read my mind (*though I sometimes wish they could*), so I have to tell them, *often more than once*, what I need from them.

For example, people have no idea what to do when I start spasming, and often their first instinct is to do exactly what I would rather they not do: make a big deal about the fact that I am spasming. I speak up and tell people that if I start spasming and they don't know how to relax me, the best thing they can do is keep talking with me and distract me from the pain. I also tell them that if I stop moving, don't assume that there's a problem. Sometimes I just want to take a moment to collect my thoughts or catch my breath. The best thing for me is to keep the conversation going so I am distracted.

I believe in speaking up about consumer issues, not just health issues. If you don't speak up, how will things ever get better? Recently, my brother and I went out with Dad to a favorite Italian restaurant. We ordered mozzarella and tomatoes from the menu, but the dish came topped with prosciutto, which was not mentioned on the menu. Pork products are not hallal, so my brother and I couldn't eat that dish. The restaurant should have known better — we are regular customers. I spoke to a waiter about it. That restaurant won't make that mistake again, and we'll keep going there.

Chapter 45
Perspective

Don't take life TOO seriously; you'll never get out alive.

It's often tempting for me to escape into my head because I don't have the abilities that most people were born with. I can't just go for a stroll in the park, or grab the keys to my car and drive around to blow off steam. Because of these limitations, I seem to function as both the Ying and Yang of contradicting personas (if you're into Chinese philosophy and tangible dualities and I butchered this . . . I'm sorry; I'm not sorry. #YOLO). On the one hand, I take life very seriously; however, whenever I can, I try to be an "in the moment" person and never take life for granted. I think people are getting out of the habit of being present in the moment and enjoying the people and places around them. They are overly focused on work, social media, or what the latest "trend" is, and they forget what it means to enjoy the moment. A moment can't be shared on Twitter or Instagram; it's not something you enjoy vicariously through someone else's Facebook feed. It's something you see and feel and experience for yourself. If you are hanging out with me, I need you to be present emotionally, mentally, and physically to the best of your ability.

Chapter 46
Heroes

With the anxiety, PTSD, and depression, it's very hard for me to go on. I feel trapped, alone, and that nobody understands me. I feel like living like this can be unbearable. I have my faith, music, and people that inspire me, such as Jared Padalecki and Demi Lovato. I love Jared's TV show, *Supernatural*. While the show takes place in a world with a lot of fantasy aspects, such as paranormal predators, it is actually the most accurate presentation of my mental dynamics. It shows the kind of pain I feel. And by doing that, it eases my pain. It is amazing to watch a show that gets what you want to say and how you feel without you even saying it.

What makes it even better is that Jared has shared with the world the story of his own struggles with depression and anxiety. He launched a campaign called "Always Keep Fighting" to raise funds for people dealing with addiction, depression, self-injury, and suicide. More recently, he has evolved the campaign so its current message is "Love Yourself First/Always Keep Fighting/I Am Enough." It is great advice! His campaign has helped me because it is hard to love myself and hard to keep fighting because of the way I look. It's hard to keep fighting because of my physical limitations and the things that I have been through.

One show that has changed my life is *Speechless* on ABC. All my life, I thought it not possible for a person like me to be in show business. Now I know that while it may take longer, it is actually a possibility. *Speechless* is a family comedy about raising a child with cerebral palsy. Minnie Driver stars as the mother, and she reminds me of my mom. Michah Fowler plays the lead. His character is in some ways like me . . . mischievous yet lovable at the same time.

Demi Lovato, through her music, is also open about mental illness and bullying. She writes and speaks the truth about how it feels to suffer. She went through a very public struggle with bipolar disorder, and now she is a spokesperson for the "Be Vocal: Speak Up for Mental Health" campaign. The lyrics of most of her songs are so powerful and so moving that they help me because there is so much that I want to say. The saying "words can't describe how I feel" is so true, but her songs speak for me and to me. I am hoping that one day my music is as beautiful and strong as hers.

Both of these celebrities are very strong for admitting their pain in such a public way. It is not easy to go through it, much less announce it to the world. Knowing that there are celebrities that go through these struggles and not only persevere but try to help is very comforting.

Chapter 47
Invitation: Ask Me!

Now that you know a little about how different my body is from yours and how complicated my life experience can be, you may be inclined to be super-cautious when you interact with me. Don't be that way. Ask me questions. I'm not all that delicate. I survived a terrible car crash, so I can probably survive your question. My body may have some unusual limitations, but my brain and heart and personality are at least full-size and full-power — and maybe even more than that.

I might tell you that your question is none of your business or I'm not comfortable answering that. I might give you a sarcastic answer. But I'll probably be straightforward with you. Sure, you don't know much about me. But if you ask sincerely, I'll educate you. In fact, I'll start the process right now by answering three questions you might have.

Chapter 48
Who Am I?

The first thing you would probably notice about me is that I am in a wheelchair, attached to a machine, my vent. I am quadriplegic: my head is just fine (this is debatable), and I have no control of my body below my neck. This has to do with the level of my spinal cord injury. Being in a wheelchair and having to rely on other people is ANNOYING AS HELL.

The second thing you would probably notice about me is my voice. I, for the most part, will speak up, in part to be sure that you keep yourself at a distance and don't bump into me, my chair, or my tray — any of which would be painful for me. I'm not shy. I'll tell you where I want you to be and what I want you to do. If I had control of my arms and hands, I would probably snap my fingers or clap my hands when I give marching orders. But I don't have control of those parts of my body, so I underscore my orders with a couple of clucks of my tongue. I'm impatient by nature. I'm not rude; my comments are always made with a smile. My friends can tell how good I feel about someone by how I treat them: the closer a person is to me, the more likely I am to insult them in a friendly way. I've even had friends who thought I was mad at them because I didn't insult them! I speak quickly; if you're not from the New York–New Jersey area, you might want me to slow down a bit.

If there were a Venn diagram with three circles — one for people with severe spinal cord injuries; one for people who experience mental illnesses; one for modern, young women — you'd find me in the small space where those circles overlap. And, if you wanted to, you could add a few more circles to the diagram — one for people of Islamic faith; one for people of Italian heritage; one for people who say what's on their mind without a lot of editing — and I'd still be at the intersection of all of those sets. *(Note to my former math teachers: Despite what you may have thought, I was listening and learning in your class.)*

There are also a few circles you could draw where I would be the only person who belonged inside. As far as I know, I am by far the youngest person to survive the kind of spinal cord injury I experienced. My injury happened when I was two years old. You could call a circle "people who can sing and act while relying on a vent to breathe," and, again, I think I would be the only person who belonged in the circle.

The point is that while I can be representative of, and speak for, various groups of people, I myself am unique. There is only one of me. I have my own attitudes, my own personality, my own mannerisms. I am smart and learn quickly but am not necessarily inclined to the typical classroom experience. I am extremely empathetic and able to feel the pains that others experience, but I don't hesitate to make the people around me do my bidding. I have to be this way because of all the things that I cannot do. I am a bundle of contradictions, just like any other person.

Chapter 49
Why Did I Write This Book?

I had several reasons for writing this book. The immediately obvious reasons are that I have something to say and I want to be heard.

Above and beyond that, I have an intense need to be helpful, to somehow help other people. By telling the story of my trials and tribulations, I hope that I can inspire other people who have suffered similar setbacks. I also hope this book will help "typical" people understand what injured people face and that no matter how challenged someone is, they remain a person full of emotions, thoughts, hopes, and dreams. They may be harder to communicate with, but they deserve your attention.

And beneath those motivations, there's something more. When I was two years old, I was in a rehab unit with other children who had serious injuries or illnesses. Throughout my life, I found that there were times when some of the other patients would need help but would be unable or unwilling to ask for it. So I felt and feel an incessant need to speak up for them. For example, I have a friend who can't speak, and I remember calling out to the nurse, "Amanda's line is off. Reconnect her so she can breathe." Speaking up for someone who can't speak just felt right to me, even at that young age. Since then, I have had many opportunities to speak for people. While this book can't speak for everyone in a specific situation, I hope it can spread the understanding that even when something isn't said, it doesn't mean that there isn't something that should have been said.

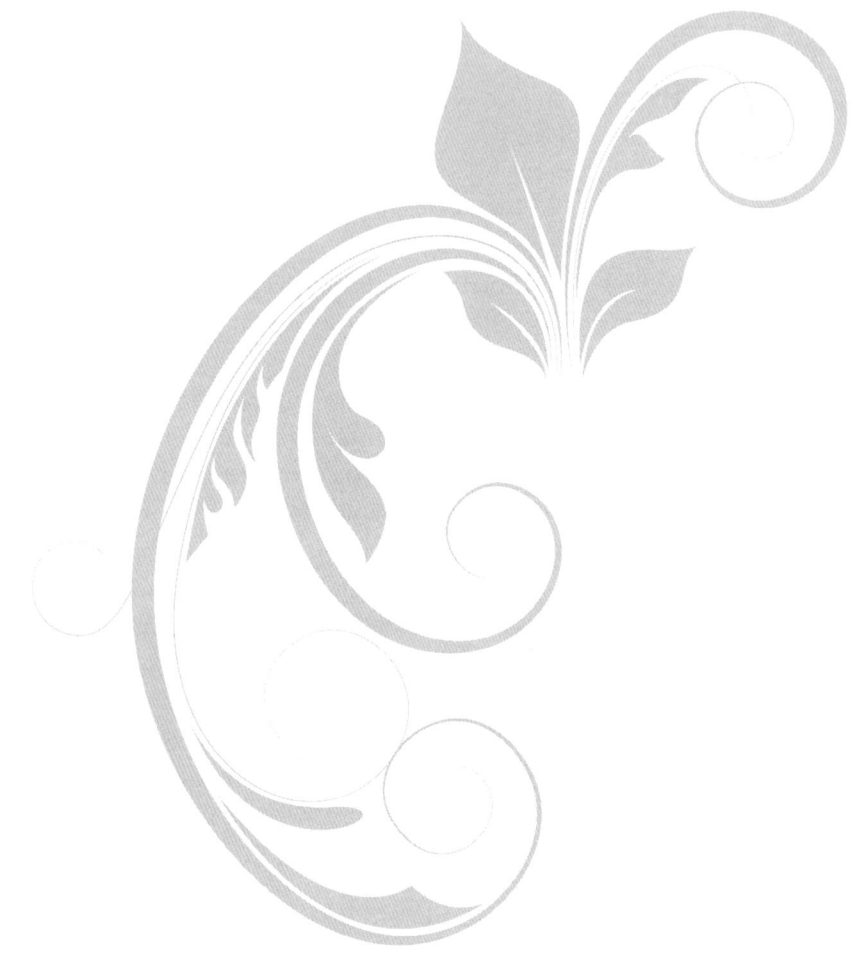

Chapter 50
How Did I Write This Book?

If you've been paying attention, you might have started to wonder how someone who is quadriplegic could write a book. The answer is that I use a variety of methods. First of all, I type by using special equipment that responds to "puffs and sips" — exhales and inhales — on a custom-designed straw. This is as tough and as tedious as it sounds. Probably even tougher because I have severely reduced lung power as a result of my injury. Each word is a trial. Each sentence is a long ordeal. *This should give you an idea as to how motivated I was to write this book* since it takes a lot of strength for me to type. Of course, when I type with my straw, my mother gets frustrated just watching me.

Obviously, I can often work more efficiently if I have someone helping me *(the story of my life)*. Out of all the ways there are for me to write, dictating to someone who types for me and reviewing the text on my Apple TV is the easiest. When I am skipping around and telling somebody what to do while making whatever changes and corrections are necessary, an assistant makes things easier. We put the document up on the big screen on my television in front of me.

Every now and then, someone sees how hard it is for me to type and asks me why I don't use voice recognition software. The answer is simple: I have tried Dragon NaturallySpeaking, a popular voice recognition program, and as much as I love the idea of typing via voice recognition software, it is not as simple as it seems. It requires a lot of patience. I talk fast because my mind races very fast and I come from a fast-speaking family. The software is also sensitive to noise, and my vent creates a lot of background noise. I have found that it takes longer to correct and fix the resulting document than it would have taken for me to type the document with my straw. *Annoyingly, my younger brother seems to have no problems using Dragon. (Ha Ha)*

Chapter 51
Forgiving

Why have I survived and been able to develop my voice? I think that God, Allah, has a special plan in mind for me. I don't know what that plan is, but I do know that I want to help people, I think by sharing the lessons that I learned. I may be a young adult, but there are still many lessons and challenges that I am overcoming or at least trying.

One of the biggest and most difficult challenges that I'm trying to overcome is forgiveness. For years, I have been asking myself, "What would I say to the driver who did this to me?" Each day I have a different answer because it really depends on my mood and what's going on in my life. I think I am finally ready to come up with an answer.

I am not happy that I am like this, but as I said earlier, I can manage. I learned forgiveness. I am not one to forgive and forget that easily, but I finally think I can forgive him. Some days, when my depression is really bad, I ask, "What did I do to deserve this?" But if I really believe in Allah, I won't let this stop me from doing what I love to do. I don't know anything other than this injury. This is my life. Yes, I would love to get up and walk or have normal human experiences, but I am trying to accept that it is not for me. When you have depression or some sort of mental illness or a lot of frustration going on, you get angry and you start hurting. I try not to let it stop me and try not to be angry. I think the best thing to say is that I am more hurt than angry. This goes for everybody, although it's not as easy as it seems, but you will feel so much better if you learn to forgive and let go.

One way to make it easier to forgive and let go is when I pay it forward and give back. By giving it back, no matter how you do it, it will help you because it shows that you are not the only one who is suffering. There is so much that needs to be done in terms of spinal cord injuries and mental illness, and I feel that by me spreading the word, eventually the outcome will be very rewarding. Focusing on giving is much more uplifting than focusing on your own trauma.

Chapter 52
My Destiny

I believe it's my destiny, my job, to speak for those who are voiceless or are afraid to speak. I want to help the world understand that there is more than what the outside shows, and that the real beauty is within. So I am hoping that this book has helped you, whether you have a physical disability or mental disability or you are just struggling in one way or another. After all, we are all human; we all have the same needs and emotions. Alhamdulillah, we are managing and are still trying to manage. *If I can do it, you can do it too. And hey, we are the only ones who know our bodies.*